Hearing

AN INTRODUCTION & PRACTICAL GUIDE

Hearing

AN INTRODUCTION & PRACTICAL GUIDE

James R. Tysome MBBS, MA, PhD, FRCS(ORL-HNS)
Consultant ENT and Skull Base Surgeon
Addenbrooke's Hospital
Cambridge University Hospitals NHS Foundation Trust
Cambridge, UK

Rahul G. Kanegaonkar FRCS(ORL-HNS)
Consultant ENT Surgeon
Medway NHS Foundation Trust
Visiting Professor in Otorhinolaryngology
Canterbury Christ Church University
Canterbury, UK

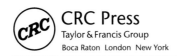

CRC Press
Taylor & Francis Group
Boca Raton London New York

CRC Press is an imprint of the
Taylor & Francis Group, an **informa** business

CRC Press
Taylor & Francis Group
6000 Broken Sound Parkway NW, Suite 300
Boca Raton, FL 33487-2742

Printed on acid-free paper
Version Date: 20151012

International Standard Book Number-13: 978-1-4987-0864-7 (Paperback)

Visit the Taylor & Francis Web site at
http://www.taylorandfrancis.com

and the CRC Press Web site at
http://www.crcpress.com

To
Laura, George, Henry and Max
and
Dipalee, Amee and Deven

CONTENTS

PREFACE

Hearing is essential for normal communication. The ear is a highly developed and sensitive organ able to detect sound waves with an amplitude of just 20 μPa, 2×10^{-10} times atmospheric pressure. The sound wave displaces the basilar membrane by only 0.2 nm, although this is amplified significantly by contraction of the outer hair cells. We are able to localise sound with surprising accuracy, detecting time differences as small as the time it takes sound to pass from one ear and reach the other. Central processing of sound in the auditory cortex allows us to distinguish speech despite background noise.

Hearing loss is a common problem affecting 40% of people over 50 and 70% when over 70. It is a sad fact that the mean time from patients noticing hearing impairment to seeking help is 10 years in the developed world. While newborn hearing screening has made a significant difference in the early diagnosis of congenital profound hearing loss in countries where it is compulsory, thus facilitating cochlear implantation prior to the development of speech and language to improve outcomes, we are still only implanting a small proportion of adults who would benefit from cochlear implantation.

This book provides the reader with an introduction to hearing. It contains the basic knowledge required to understand hearing in terms of anatomy and physiology as well as a practical guide on how to assess and manage patients with all aspects of hearing loss.

James R. Tysome and Rahul G. Kanegaonkar

CONTRIBUTORS

Patrick Axon MD, FRCS(ORL-HNS)
Consultant Otoneurological and Skull Base Surgeon
Addenbrooke's Hospital
Cambridge University Hospitals NHS Foundation Trust
Cambridge, UK

David M. Baguley PhD, MBA
Consultant Clinical Scientist, Head of Service: Audiology/Hearing
    Implants
Visiting Professor, Anglia Ruskin University
Cambridge University Hospitals NHS Foundation Trust
Cambridge, UK

Mahmood F. Bhutta FRCS, DPhil
Clinical Lecturer, University College London Ear Institute
Specialist Registrar, Royal National Throat, Nose and Ear Hospital
University College London Ear Institute
London, UK

Stephen Broomfield MBChB, FRCS(ORL-HNS)
ENT Consultant
University Hospitals Bristol NHS Foundation Trust
Bristol, UK

Philip J. Clamp BMBCh, MA, DOHNS, FRCS(ORL-HNS)
Consultant in Otolaryngology
University Hospitals Bristol NHS Foundation Trust
Bristol, UK

Steve Connor MBChB(Hons), MRCP, FRCR
King's College Hospital NHS Foundation Trust
London, UK

Neil Donnelly MSc(Hons), MBBS, FRCS(ORL-HNS)
Consultant ENT Surgeon
Addenbrooke's Hospital
Cambridge University Hospitals NHS Foundation Trust
Cambridge, UK

Simon R.M. Freeman MBChB, BSc(Hons), MPhil, FRCS(ORL-HNS)
Consultant Otolaryngologist and Skull Base Surgeon
Manchester Royal Infirmary
Central Manchester University Hospitals NHS Foundation Trust
Manchester, UK

Richard K. Gurgel MD
Assistant Professor, Division of Otolaryngology – Head and
    Neck Surgery
University of Utah School of Medicine
Salt Lake City, USA

William P.L. Hellier FRCS(ORL-HNS)
Consultant ENT Surgeon, University Hospital Southampton
Honorary Senior Lecturer, University of Southampton
Southampton, UK

Elizabeth Hough MA, MSc, PhD
Clinical Scientist (Audiology)
Addenbrooke's Hospital
Cambridge University Hospitals NHS Foundation Trust
Cambridge, UK

Richard Irving MD, FRCS(ORL-HNS)
Consultant in Otology, Neurotology and Skull Base Surgery
Queen Elizabeth Hospital Birmingham
Birmingham Children's Hospital
Birmingham, UK

Rahul G. Kanegaonkar FRCS(ORL-HNS)
Consultant ENT Surgeon
Medway NHS Foundation Trust
Visiting Professor in Otorhinolaryngology, Canterbury Christ Church
    University
Canterbury, UK

Bruno M.R. Kenway BMedSci, BMBS, DOHNS, FRCS(ORL-HNS)
Addenbrooke's Hospital
Cambridge University Hospitals NHS Foundation Trust
Cambridge, UK

Richard D. Knight PhD, MSc
Clinical Scientist (Audiology)
Head of Vestibular Service
Cambridge University Hospitals NHS Foundation Trust
Cambridge, UK

H.P.M. Kunst MD, PhD
Otologist/Skull Base Surgeon
Radboud University Medical Center
Nijmegen, The Netherlands

Jeremy A. Lavy FRCS(Eng), FRCS(ORL-HNS)
Consultant ENT Surgeon
Royal National ENT Hospital
London, UK

Ruth V. Lloyd MBChB, FRCS
ENT Consultant
Pembury Hospital
Tunbridge Wells, UK

Simon Lloyd MBBS, BSc(Hons), MPhil, FRCS(ORL-HNS)
Consultant ENT Surgeon
Central Manchester University Hospitals NHS Foundation Trust
    (Manchester Royal Infirmary)
Salford Royal NHS Foundation Trust (Salford Royal Hospital)
Manchester, UK

Thomas P.C. Martin MD, FRCS(ORL-HNS)
Consultant ENT Surgeon
Worcester Royal Hospital
Worcester, UK

Don J. McFerran MA, MB, BChir, MA, FRCS(ORL-HNS)
Consultant ENT Surgeon
Colchester Hospital University NHS Foundation Trust
Colchester, UK

Peter Monksfield FRCS(ORL-HNS)
Consultant Otolaryngologist and Skull Base Surgeon
University Hospitals Birmingham
Birmingham, UK

Victoria H. Parfect BSc, MSc, CS
Addenbrooke's Hospital
Cambridge University Hospitals NHS Foundation Trust
Cambridge, UK

Nicholas A. Quinn MD
Division of Otolaryngology – Head and Neck Surgery
University of Utah School of Medicine
Salt Lake City, USA

Nick Saunders FRCS(ORL-HNS)
Consultant ENT Surgeon
Brighton and Sussex University Hospitals Trust
Western Sussex Hospitals NHS Foundation Trust
Brighton, UK

Holger H. Sudhoff FRCS(Lon), FRCPath
Department of Otolaryngology, Head and Neck Surgery
Bielefeld Academic Teaching Hospital
Muenster University
Bielefeld, Germany

Aaron Trinidade FRCS(ORL-HNS)
Addenbrooke's Hospital
Cambridge University Hospitals NHS Foundation Trust
Cambridge, UK

James R. Tysome MBBS, MA, PhD, FRCS(ORL-HNS)
Consultant ENT and Skull Base Surgeon
Addenbrooke's Hospital
Cambridge University Hospitals NHS Foundation Trust
Cambridge, UK

Max Whittaker MBBS, MRCS, DOHNS
Specialist Registrar in Otolaryngology
Kent, Sussex and Surrey Rotation
London, UK

Ian M. Winter BSc, D.Phil
The Physiological Laboratory
Cambridge, UK

Maarten de Wolf MD, PhD
Fellow in Otology Neurotology and Skull Base Surgery
Queen Elizabeth Hospital Birmingham
Birmingham Children's Hospital
Birmingham, UK
Currently at Department of Otorhinolaryngology
Academic Medical Centre, Amsterdam, Netherlands

Sarah Yorke-Smith MChem, PhD, MSc
Addenbrooke's Hospital
Cambridge University Hospitals NHS Foundation Trust
Cambridge, UK

ABBREVIATIONS

ABI	auditory brainstem implant
ABR	auditory brainstem response
AIED	autoimmune inner ear disease
AOM	acute otitis media
ARTA	age-related typical audiogram
BAHA	bone-anchored hearing aid
BET	balloon Eustachian tuboplasty
BM	basilar membrane
CANS	central auditory nervous system
(C)APD	(central) auditory processing disorder
CBCT	cone beam computed tomography
CHL	conductive hearing loss
CI	cochlear implant
CNS	central nervous system
COME	chronic otitis media with effusion
CROS	contralateral routing of signal
CSF	cerebrospinal fluid
CSOM	chronic suppurative otitis media
CT	computed tomography
CVC	consonant-vowel-consonant
DPOAE	distortion product otoacoustic emission
EAC	external auditory canal
ET	Eustachian tube
ETD	Eustachian tube dysfunction
FMT	floating mass transducer
HA	hearing aid
HRTF	head-related transfer function
HSP	heat shock protein
IC	inferior colliculus
IHCs	inner hair cells
LDL	loudness discomfort level
LSO	lateral superior olive
MEI	middle ear implant
MNTB	medial nucleus of the trapezoid body
MRI	magnetic resonance imaging
MRL	minimum response level
MSO	medial superior olive
NF2	neurofibromatosis type 2
NIHL	noise-induced hearing loss
OHCs	outer hair cells
OM	otitis media

OME	otitis media with effusion
PORP	partial ossicular replacement prosthesis
PTA	pure tone audiometry
rAOM	recurrent acute otitis media
REM	real ear measurement
SC	superior colliculus
SNHI	sensorineural hearing impairment
SNHL	sensorineural hearing loss
SOC	superior olive complex
SRS	stereotactic radiosurgery
SSNHL	sudden sensorineural hearing loss
TEOAE	transient evoked otoacoustic emission
TM	tympanic membrane
TMM	tubomanometry
TORP	total ossicular replacement prosthesis
VRA	visual reinforcement audiometry

I

BASIC SCIENCE OF HEARING

1

THE ANATOMY OF HEARING

Rahul G. Kanegaonkar & Max Whittaker

Contents

INTRODUCTION

The ear is divided into three separate but functionally-related subunits. The outer ear consists of the pinna and external auditory canal (EAC) bounded medially by the lateral surface of the tympanic membrane (TM). The middle ear contains the ossicular chain, which spans the middle ear cleft and allows acoustic energy to be transferred from the TM to the oval window and then into the cochlea of the inner ear. This elaborate mechanism has evolved to overcome the loss of acoustic energy that occurs when transferring sound from one medium to another (impedance mismatch), in this case from air to fluid.

OUTER EAR

PINNA

▐ Embryology

The pinna develops from six mesodermal conden-
sations, the hillocks of His (**Figure 1.1**), during the
sixth week of embryological development. Three
arise from each of the first and second branchial
arches on either side of the first pharyngeal groove.
These fuse and rotate to produce an elaborate but
remarkably consistent structure. The first branchial arch gives rise to the tragus, helix and cymba
conchae, whereas the conchal bowl, antitragus
and antihelix, and hence the bulk of the pinna, are
derived from the second arch. While a rudimen-
tary pinna is present at 60 days, it is fully formed at
4 months. Failure of fusion may result in an acces-
sory auricle or preauricular sinus, while failure

of development of the antihelix (from the fourth
hillock) may result in a protruding or 'Bat' ear.

▐ Anatomy

The pinna consists largely of elastic cartilage over
which the skin is tightly adherent (**Figure 1.2**).
The cartilage is dependent on the overlying perichondrium for its nutritional support, therefore
separation of this layer by a haematoma, abscess
or inflammation secondary to piercing or trauma
may result in cartilage necrosis and permanent
deformity (cauliflower ear). The lobule, in contrast,
is a fibrofatty skin tag. The complex sensory nerve
supply of the pinna is reflected in its embryological
origin (see **Table 1.1**).

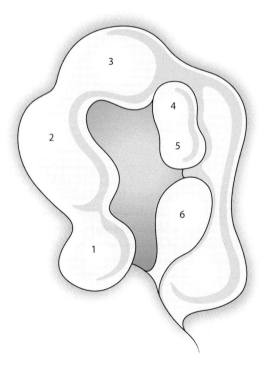

Figure 1.1. Development of the pinna at approximately 7 weeks of age. The six hillocks of His are
fusing to form two folds, which will later fuse superiorly.

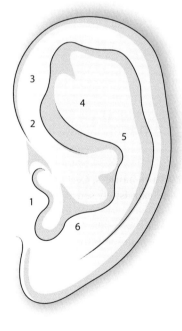

Figure 1.2. The external ear. The adult auricle
with the derivatives of the six hillocks of His
numbered.

Table 1.1. The sensory nerve supply of the pinna.

Nerve	Derivation	Region supplied
Greater auricular	Cervical plexus C2/C3	Medial surface and posterior part of lateral surface of pinna
Lesser occipital	Cervical plexus C2	Superior portion of medial surface
Auricular	Vagus	Concha and antihelix
Auriculotemporal	Mandibular division of trigeminal nerve	Tragus, crus of the helix and adjacent helix
Facial		Supplies root of concha

EXTERNAL AUDITORY CANAL

▮ Embryology

The EAC develops from the upper part of the first pharyngeal groove. Initially funnel shaped, this tube deepens and widens by ectodermal proliferation to briefly come into contact with the endoderm of the first pharyngeal pouch. Mesenchymal infiltration then separates these two layers to eventually form the fibrous middle layer of the TM.

▮ Anatomy

The EAC is a tortuous passage approximately 2.5 cm in length that directs sound from the conchal bowl to the TM. The skin of the lateral third of the EAC is thick, hair-bearing, contains ceruminous glands and is adherent to the underlying fibrocartilage. In contrast, the skin of the medial two-thirds is thin, hairless, tightly bound to underlying bone and exquisitely sensitive.

The auriculotemporal and greater auricular nerves largely provide the sensory nerve supply of the canal. There are minor contributions from the facial nerve (hence vesicles arise on the posterolateral surface of the canal in Ramsay Hunt syndrome) and Arnold's nerve, a branch of the vagus nerve (provoking the cough reflex when stimulated during microsuction). The squamous epithelium of the TM and ear canal is unique and is worthy of consideration. The superficial layer of keratin of the skin of the ear is shed laterally during maturation. This produces an escalator mechanism, allowing clearance of debris out of the canal. Disruption of this mechanism may result in debris accumulation and may predispose to recurrent infections (otitis externa) or erosion of the ear canal as seen in keratitis obturans.

The TM is continuous with the posterior wall of the ear canal and consists of three layers: laterally a squamous epithelial layer; a middle layer of collagen fibres; and a medial surface lined with respiratory epithelium continuous with the middle ear (**Figure 1.3**). The TM is divided into the pars tensa and the pars flaccida, or attic (**Figure 1.3**). These differ both structurally and functionally.

The collagen fibres of the middle layer of the pars tensa are arranged as lateral radial fibres and medial circumferential fibres that distort the membrane. As a result, the pars tensa 'billows' laterally from the malleus. In contrast, the collagen fibres of the pars flaccida are randomly scattered and this section is relatively flat. While the surface area of the TM of an adult is approximately 80 mm^2, the pars tensa accounts for 55 mm^2. Unlike the pars flaccida, the pars tensa buckles when presented with sound, conducting acoustic energy to the ossicular chain. Interestingly, high frequency sounds preferentially alter the posterior half of the TM, while low frequency sounds alter

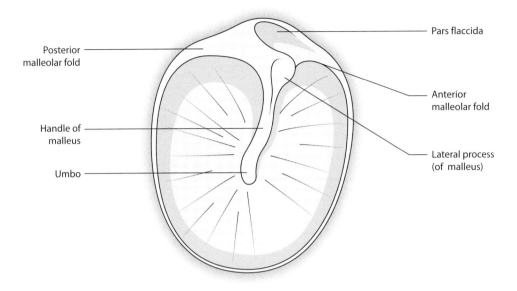

Figure 1.3. The tympanic membrane.

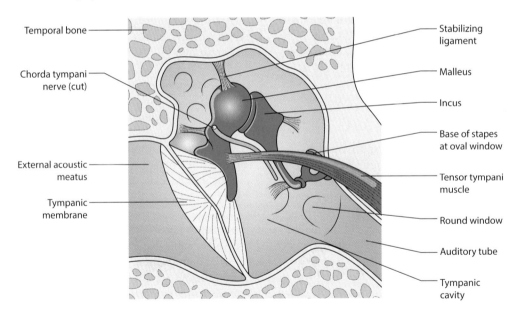

Figure 1.4. The middle ear.

the anterior half. Furthermore, the arrangement of the EAC and TM as a blind ending tube acts as a resonator. This effect increases sound pressure by up to 12 dB within the frequency region around 3 kHz, with particular implications for the perception of speech.

The handle and lateral process of the malleus are embedded within the TM and are clearly visible on otoscopy. The long process of the incus is also commonly seen, although the heads of the ossicles are hidden behind the scutum superiorly (**Figure 1.4**).

MIDDLE EAR

The middle ear is an irregular air filled space that communicates with the nasopharynx via the Eustachian tube (**Figure 1.4**). Chewing, swallowing and yawning result in transient opening of the tube, allowing air to pass into the middle ear cleft. In children, Eustachian tube dysfunction is common, and may result in negative middle ear pressure, recurrent otitis media or middle ear effusion.

▌ Anatomy

The malleus articulates via a synovial joint with the incus, which in turn similarly articulates with the stapes. The ossicular chain is suspended within the middle ear space by a number of ligaments and mucosal folds (**Figure 1.4**). In addition, ossicular vibrations are modified by the actions of the tendon of tensor tympani, innervated by a branch of the mandibular division of the trigeminal nerve and inserting into the neck of the malleus, and the stapedius tendon, innervated by a branch of the facial nerve and inserting into the neck of stapes (**Figure 1.4**).

The irregular surface of the medial wall of the right middle ear is illustrated in **Figure 1.5**. The majority is made up by the promontory, a protrusion of the basal turn of the cochlea. The stapes footplate lies in a groove between this prominence and the facial nerve.

Acoustic energy is conducted by the middle ear ossicles and transferred to the cochlea through the stapes footplate at the oval window. Known as the middle ear transformer mechanism, this process is optimised by the factors listed in **Table 1.2**.

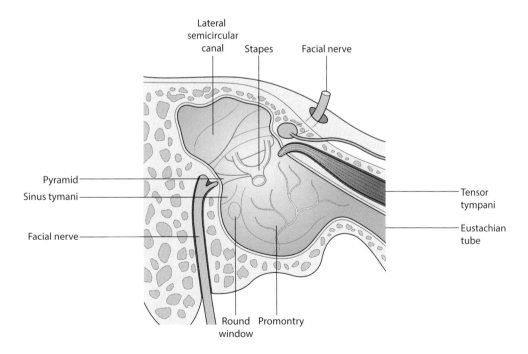

Figure 1.5. The medial wall of the middle ear.

Table 1.2. Factors optimising the middle ear transformer.

Hydraulic ratio	Tympanic membrane:stapes footplate	14:1
Lever arm ratio	Malleus:incus	1.3:1
Total		18.2:1

From: McDonogh M (1986) The middle ear transformer mechanism: man versus mouse. *J Laryngol Otol* **100(1):**15–20.

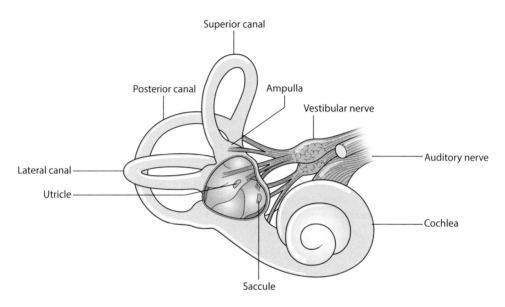

Figure 1.6. The inner ear.

INNER EAR

The inner ear is comprised of the cochlea and the peripheral vestibular apparatus (**Figure 1.6**). While the peripheral vestibular apparatus is dedicated to detecting angular and linear acceleration and static head tilt, the cochlea is devoted to hearing. Both of these structures consist of a membranous labyrinth encased within the bony labyrinth of the otic capsule.

Cochlea

▌ Embryology

The inner ear structures develop from a pair of otic placodes, two thickenings of ectoderm flanking the neural tube, apparent from the fourth gestational week. Induced by fibroblast growth factors, the placodes progressively sink into the underlying mesenchyme to form the otic cups and eventually otocysts. The complex three-dimensional structure of the mature inner ear is achieved through a process of regionalisation under the influence of multiple diffusible factors including Wnt and

Sonic Hedgehog. Neuroblasts delaminate from the otocyst to form the cochleovestibular ganglion, which eventually innervates the sensory domains. The production of hair cells within the organ of Corti occurs during weeks 11–12 and is regulated by expression of the Atoh1 gene through a process of lateral inhibition with neighbouring cells. Hair cell production progresses from the cochlear apex to the base, while cell maturation and innervation paradoxically occurs from base to apex. During this process, neural crest cells migrate along the auditory nerve and invade the cochleovestibular ganglion, giving rise to satellite cells and Schwann cells, which eventually myelinate auditory nerve fibres. Cochlear maturation is complete by birth, although the onset of function is thought to occur between weeks 18 and 20 (**Figure 1.7**).

▌ Anatomy

The cochlea is a two-and-three-quarters turn snail shell that houses the organ of Corti (**Figure 1.8**). When uncoiled it is approximately 35 mm in length. In cross-section it is separated into three distinct chambers: the scala vestibuli and scala tympani filled with perilymph and joined at the helicotrema, and the scala media filled with endolymph. The perilymphatic space is in continuity with the subarachnoid space, connected by the cochlear aqueduct, and as such its ionic composition bears resemblance to CSF, with comparable low concentrations of potassium. In contrast, the endolymphatic system, while connected to the endolymphatic sac by the vestibular aqueduct, is closed and is rich in potassium. In the cochlea this ionic gradient is crucial in achieving the endocochlear potential necessary for the normal physiological function of hair cells.

Acoustic energy transmitted via the oval window into the cochlear fluids causes vibration of the basilar membrane, with maximal deflection at frequency-specific regions. A second cochlear fenestration, the round window, acts as a pressure relief port allowing for transmission of basilar membrane travelling waves through the perilymph. The cochlea is tonotopic with high frequency sounds detected at the basal turn and low frequency sounds detected at the apex. The basilar membrane itself is partly responsible for this property, being narrow and stiff near the base and becoming progressively wider and more flexible towards the apex. Vibrations result in hair bundle deflection and depolarisation of inner hair cells in corresponding regions. This single row of cells within the organ of Corti forms the main source of sensory input. Neuronal impulses are transmitted by afferent auditory nerve fibres, whose cell bodies lie in the spiral ganglion, and beyond which form the cochlear branch of the vestibulocochlear nerve. In contrast, the three rows of outer hair cells, predominantly innervated by efferent fibres, are responsible for frequency tuning and amplification within the cochlea.

Cochlear blood supply is derived from the spiral modiolar artery, a branch of the labyrinthine artery. Blood is drained via the spiral modiolar vein.

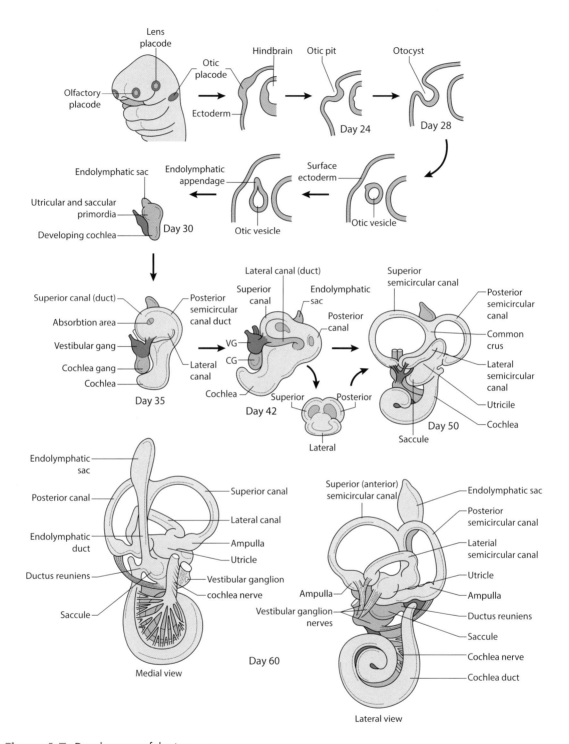

Figure 1.7. Development of the inner ear.

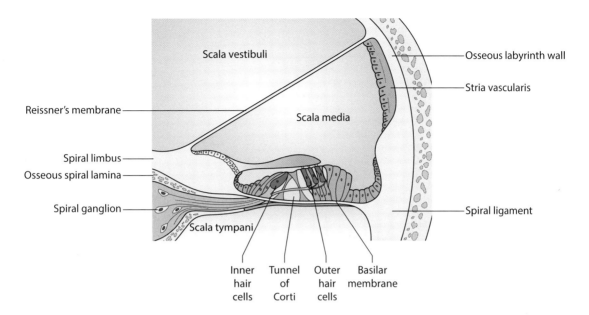

Figure 1.8. The organ of Corti.

2

PHYSIOLOGY OF HEARING
Basic principles of audiology

Ian M. Winter

Contents

INTRODUCTION

The auditory pathway can be divided into the peripheral auditory system, comprising the ear and the auditory nerve, and the central auditory system, comprising the nuclei and pathways from the cochlear nucleus to the auditory cortex. The ear has been classically divided into three parts: outer (pinna and external auditory meatus); middle (tympanic membrane [TM], ossicles and middle ear cavity); and inner (cochlea [includes the vestibular apparatus]) (**Figure 2.1**).

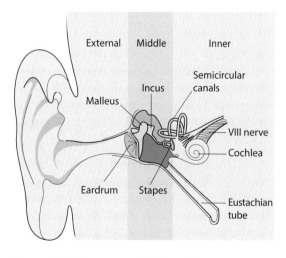

Figure 2.1. The outer, middle and inner ear.

OUTER (EXTERNAL) EAR

The external ear is comprised of the pinna and the external auditory canal (EAC). The EAC acts as an open-ended tube and has resonant peaks (predictable from its 2–3 cm length in humans) that coincide with the frequencies (2–4 kHz) important to speech. The pinna is able to assist in sound localisation by modifying the spectra of sounds in a space-dependent manner. In humans, the pressure transformation from free field to the TM, often referred to as a head-related transfer function (HRTF), contains direction-dependent notches above ~5 kHz. It has been shown that these spectral notches provide a cue for sound localisation, particularly in the vertical plane (elevation). Humans can quite quickly (a few weeks) reinterpret the relationship between cues provided by HRTFs and direction in space. For instance, when moulds are fitted to the external ear (disrupting the ability of a listener to make judgements about elevation) listeners learn to associate new spectral cues with direction in space. Remarkably, listeners could localise just as well immediately after removal of the earmould. This suggests that multiple representations of auditory space can co-exist.[1]

MIDDLE EAR

The functions of the middle ear include (1) impedance matching between air and cochlear fluids, (2) protection from loud sounds, including own vocalisations and (3) anti-masking of high frequency sounds by low frequency sounds, particularly at high sound levels. The middle ear muscles are the smallest skeletal muscles in the human body. They serve to dampen the vibrations of the ossicles (malleus, incus and stapes), thereby reducing the acoustic signal that reaches the ears. They contract about 100 ms after exposure to a loud sound and also before a person vocalises, attenuating low frequencies more than high.

INNER EAR

As far as hearing is concerned, the cochlea is the main structure of interest in the inner ear. The cochlea acts as an acoustic prism by decomposing the acoustic signal into its component frequencies. Although coiled like a snail shell, the cochlea can be viewed functionally as a straight tube compartmentalised longitudinally by the three scalae: vestibule, tympani and media. The scala media contains the organ of Corti, which is responsible for transducing the acoustic stimulus. When the stapes vibrates at the oval window, the incompressible fluids in the cochlea vibrate, causing the round window to bulge outwards. This fluid movement sets into motion the basilar membrane (BM), which is narrower and stiffer near its base than its apical end and therefore vibrates maximally for high frequency sounds near the basal end and maximally for low frequency sounds near its apex. The frequencies are said to be mapped out tonotopically along its length, with equal increments in distance corresponding to roughly equal increments in logarithmic frequency. Recent results obtained in animals with good hearing have shown the BM to be very sharply tuned – as sharp as that measured in auditory nerve fibres.

Ultimately the cochlear vibrations are transduced by hair cells (**Figure 2.2**). The one row of inner hair cells (IHCs) contains ~3,000 hair cells along the cochlear partition. There are approximately three rows of outer hair cells (OHCs), totalling ~11,000. The majority of auditory nerve fibres (90%) synapse

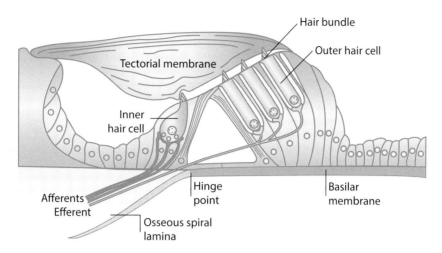

Figure 2.2. The hair cells and neural innervation pattern in the cat cochlea. A similar pattern is thought to exist for most mammals. Of principal interest are the large synaptic endings on the outer hair cells, which are from the medial olivocochlear system, and the type 1 auditory nerve fibres contacting the inner hair cells. Note that the fibres are thinner on the modiolar side of the inner hair cells and are thought to have low spontaneous discharge rate. (Adapted from Liberman MC, Dodds LW, Pierce S (1990) Afferent and efferent innervation of the cat cochlea: quantitative analysis with light and electron microscopy. *J Comp Neurol* **301:**443–460.)

with the IHCs and are known as type I fibres. The remaining 10% (type II) contact the OHCs. Type II fibres are unmyelinated and contact many OHCs. In contrast, between 10 and 20 type I fibres connect with each IHC.

Normal cochlear function is dependent on an active, mechanical feedback system. It is now widely believed that the OHCs are the agents of this feedback system, as a reduction in the responsiveness of OHCs results in a change in the response of IHCs. In addition, the ear can emit sounds, which are termed otoacoustic emissions. Otoacoustic emissions may be evoked by sound or occur spontaneously.

◼ Transduction in hair cells

In hair cells, physiological displacement of the stereocilia is caused by either a relative movement between the reticular lamina and the tectorial membrane (in the case of OHCs) or by the flow of endolymph over the cilia (in the case of IHCs). The mechanical gating of the transducer channels is thought to be controlled by tip-links, which connect the stereocilia. Transduction in hair cells is extremely fast and probably takes place at the tips of the stereocilia. If the stereocilia are stretched towards the tallest stereocilia, the probability of mechanically-gated channels opening increases; if they are stretched away from the tallest stereocilia, the probability of them closing increases. The transducer current is carried by K^+ ions, the driving force for which is entirely electrical. (**Note:** The predominant cation in the endolymph is K^+). The resting membrane potential of the hair cell (–60 mV), coupled with the large endolymphatic potential (~+80 mV), gives a total ionic gradient of 140 mV. The composition of the scala media's endolymphatic fluid is largely controlled by the stria vascularis. A reduction in the magnitude of the endocochlear potential results in a loss of auditory thresholds that can mimic that seen in presbyacusis.

In summary, the IHCs act to transduce the mechanical events in the cochlea to electrical events in auditory nerve fibres. They are responsible for transmitting the sensory information to the brain. The OHCs appear to actively assist the mechanics of the cochlea and are responsible for, among other things, low hearing thresholds, sharp frequency tuning, otoacoustic emissions and the dynamic range of auditory nerve fibres (see below).

AUDITORY NERVE

The output of the cochlea can be thought of as a set of parallel, overlapping, bandpass filters. Examples of a range of such filters recorded from the auditory nerve in the cat are shown in **Figure 2.3**.

Auditory nerve fibres have been divided into three groups based on their spontaneous rate (SR), which is defined as the discharge rate of an auditory neuron in the absence of controlled acoustic stimulation. Fibres with the lowest thresholds (the most sensitive) have the highest SRs, whereas those with the highest thresholds (least sensitive) have the lowest SRs. Those with intermediate thresholds have intermediate SRs. An auditory nerve fibre's threshold determines its dynamic range. Low threshold fibres have the narrowest dynamic range, high threshold fibres have the widest dynamic range (**Figure 2.4**).

▋ Temporal coding

Low frequency auditory neurons discharge at preferred phases of the stimulating signal. They do not necessarily discharge once every cycle, but when they do discharge they do so at the preferred phase (**Figures 2.5A, B**). The upper limit of phase-locking is not 1,000 Hz (the upper limit of spike discharge, set by the refractory period) but rather 5,000 Hz in the cat, 3,500 Hz in the guinea pig and 8,000 Hz in the barn owl. The upper limit of phase-locking in the human auditory nerve is unknown but recent, indirect, measurements suggest it is less than the cat but greater than the guinea pig.

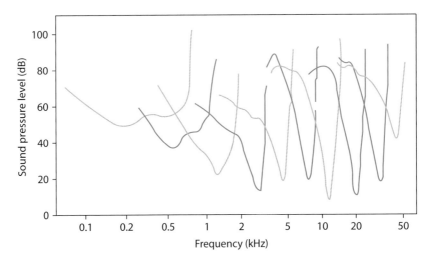

Figure 2.3. The filter shapes recorded from 10 auditory nerve fibres in the cat. Note the characteristic 'V' shape. Connecting the most sensitive point, the characteristic frequency (CF) of each filter provides a good estimate of the cat's audiogram. (Adapted from Palmer AR (1995) Neural signal processing. In: *Handbook of Perception and Cognition*. (ed. BCJ Moore) Academic, London, pp. 75–121.)

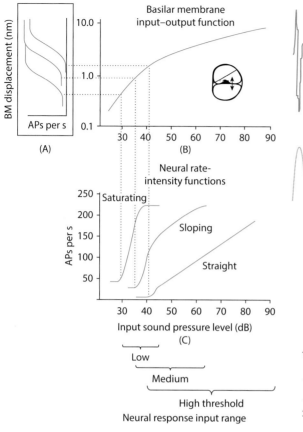

(A)

(B)

Basilar membrane
input–output function

Neural rate-
intensity functions

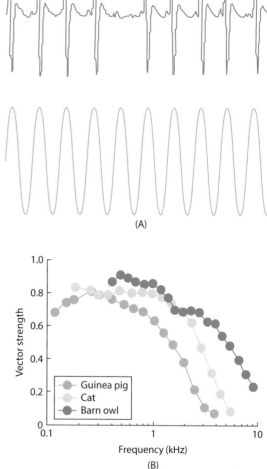

(A)

(B)

Figures 2.4A–C. How the auditory nerve fibre got its dynamic range. (A) Three sigmoidal saturating non-linearities with different thresholds. (B) The compressive growth of basilar membrane vibration with increasing sound level. (C) Dynamic ranges of individual auditory nerve fibres. Note that the lowest threshold fibres have the narrowest (saturating) dynamic range while the highest threshold fibres (characterised by low SR) have the widest (straight) dynamic range. (Adapted from Yates GK, Johnstone BM, Patuzzi RB *et al.* (1992) Mechanical preprocessing in the mammalian cochlea. *Trends Neurosci* **15(2):**57–61.)

Figures 2.5A, B. (A) Phase-locking in an auditory neuron. Top trace are action potentials (aka spikes) in response to a sinusoidal stimulus (bottom trace). The length of the scale bar is 20 ms. (B) The decline of phase-locking as a function of frequency for three commonly studied animals. A vector strength of 1.0 indicates perfect phase-locking.

By measuring the time interval between successive action potentials, it is possible to reconstruct a frequency representation of the stimulus from this phase-locked discharge. The use of temporal information for frequency coding is still a matter of debate. Temporal information is, however, used for sound localisation.

OLIVOCOCHLEAR EFFERENT SYSTEM

The olivocochlear system supplies descending fibres from the superior olive to the cochlea. It is divided into two: the lateral and medial systems. The lateral system has its cell bodies in or around the lateral superior olive (depending on the species) and the medial system has its cell bodies medial to the lateral superior olive, in the periolivary region of the superior olive. The lateral system terminates on the dendrites of the auditory nerve fibres, whereas the medial system directly contacts the OHCs. The role of the lateral olivocochlear efferent system is not known. There are three main hypotheses concerning the role of the medial olivocochlear efferent system: (1) protection from loud sounds; (2) improving detection of sounds in noise; and (3) controlling cochlear mechanics.

CENTRAL AUDITORY SYSTEM

The auditory pathway is considerably more complex than the visual pathway between receptor and cortex. The primary reason for this is presumably the need to compute the localisation of a sound source from the receptor epithelium of the cochlea, which is tonotopically organised and not spatially organised. The cochlear nucleus is an obligatory synapse for all auditory nerve fibres and has been referred to as the 'retina of the auditory system'. An enormous amount of parallel processing occurs at this point. There are cells in the cochlear nucleus specialised to preserve the timing information present in the auditory nerve input. These cells are characterised by large end-bulb of Held synapses (**Figures 2.6A, B**); these synapses are amongst the largest in the brain.

Other cells appear better suited to encode intensity and have a dynamic range considerably in excess of that found in any individual auditory nerve fibre; clearly, cells at this stage are summing information from many auditory nerve fibres. Some cells show strong lateral inhibition, analogous to that seen in the visual system and not to be confused with two-tone suppression, a non-neural phenomenon seen in the auditory nerve.

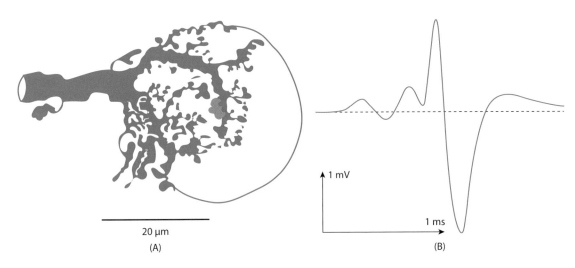

20 μm

(A)

1 mV

1 ms

(B)

Figures 2.6A, B. (A) Reconstruction of a labelled auditory nerve fibre end-bulb of Held synapse terminating on a spherical bushy cell in the cochlear nucleus. (B) The tri-phasic electrophysiological signature from these cells.

The first site of binaural convergence of the cochlear nucleus output is the superior olive complex (SOC). There are three main SOC nuclei: the lateral superior olive (LSO), the medial superior olive (MSO) and the medial nucleus of the trapezoid body (MNTB). The MSO encodes interaural time differences while the LSO encodes interaural level differences. The MNTB is the site of giant synapses from cells in the cochlear nucleus and provides inhibitory input to other nuclei in the SOC. The output of the SOC joins projections from the cochlear nucleus that form the lateral lemniscal tract. This tract terminates in the inferior colliculus. The auditory midbrain consists of the inferior colliculus (IC) and the superior colliculus (SC). Cells in the IC have been found to be spatially selective but no map

of auditory space has been found in this nucleus. In contrast, a map of auditory space does exist in the deep layers of the SC and is usually aligned with a visual map of space. It is fair to say that there is no clear idea of the functions of the mammalian auditory cortex when compared with the visual cortex. The primary auditory cortex is tonotopically organised and is bordered by one or more adjacent auditory areas.

The auditory brainstem response (ABR) is widely used in clinical settings to estimate behavioural thresholds and detect abnormalities of the auditory nerve. It is typically evoked by a short duration click (~100 µs), which yields a waveform with several peaks labelled I–V (**Figure 2.7A**). It is now

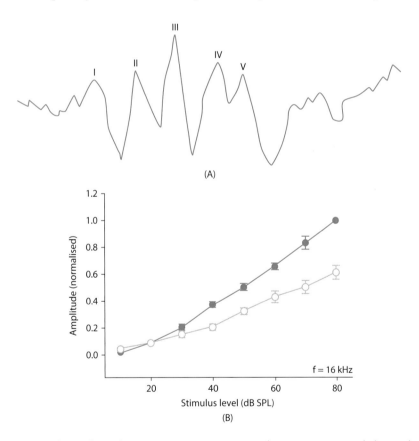

Figures 2.7A, B. (A) The auditory brainstem response measured in response to a click stimulus. (B) The normal growth in amplitude of the auditory brainstem response (filled circles) compared with the growth following acoustic over exposure (open circles) to a 16 kHz tone stimulus in the guinea pig. Note the thresholds are similar under both conditions but the growth of the auditory brainstem response with increasing sound level is much reduced following acoustic overexposure.

widely believed that waves I and II arise from the auditory nerve; indeed, the cochlear action potential is closely related to wave I. Wave III arises from the cochlear nucleus while wave IV originates in or around the SOC. Finally, wave V arises from the termination of the lateral lemniscus within the IC. The growth in amplitude of wave I has recently been used to argue that following acoustic overexposure (narrowband noise at 106 dB SPL for 2 hours), it is the low SR auditory nerve fibres that are lost selectively. **Figure 2.7B** shows the growth of amplitude of ABR wave I from the cochlea of the guinea pig before (filled squares) and after (open circles) acoustic overexposure.[2] In each condition the wave I threshold is unaltered but the rate of growth is much reduced following acoustic overexposure. A simple interpretation of these data is that the low threshold (high SR) fibres remain intact while there is a selective degeneration of high threshold (low SR) fibres. As this suprathreshold change would not normally be revealed by a routine threshold test, this phenomenon has been termed 'hidden' hearing loss.[3] The behavioural consequences of this selective neural degeneration have yet to be determined.

REFERENCES

1 Carlile S (2014) The plastic ear and perceptual relearning in auditory spatial perception. *Front Neurosci* **8(237)**:1–13.
2 Furman AC, Kujawa SG, Liberman MC (2013) Noise-induced cochlear neuropathy is selective for fibres with low spontaneous rates. *J Neurophysiol* **110**:577–586.
3 Plack CJ, Barker D, Prendergast G (2014) Perceptual consequences of "hidden" hearing loss. *Trends Hear* **18**:1–11.

FURTHER READING
Pickles JO (2012) *An Introduction to the Physiology of Hearing*, 4th edn. Emerald Press, Bingley.

II

ASSESSMENT OF HEARING

3

CLINICAL ASSESSMENT OF HEARING

Ruth V. Lloyd

Contents

INTRODUCTION

The aim of any assessment of hearing is to try to determine an individual's hearing threshold and to aid in diagnosing the cause of any hearing loss. Pure tone audiometry remains the principal method of obtaining hearing thresholds, but an understanding of the range of hearing assessments that can be performed in the clinic is invaluable. Most of these tests were developed before the advent of audiometry, but remain useful today as pure tone audiometry is not always available, and clinical tests can help assess any discrepancy between the clinical impression of a patient's hearing and their audiometry thresholds.

The main clinical tests that can be performed in the clinic or at the bedside are the 'whisper test' and tuning fork tests. Both these types of hearing assessments are subjective (i.e. they rely on the patient consciously responding to the tests). The 'whisper test' aims to give an approximate hearing threshold for each ear, and the tuning fork tests aim to help elucidate the type of hearing loss (conductive or sensorineural).

HISTORY

The history determines which tests are indicated. Important factors to determine from a patient complaining of hearing loss are:

- Is the hearing loss unilateral or bilateral?
- Associated symptoms such as tinnitus, vertigo, otalgia and otorrhoea.

- Progressive or sudden? If progressive, when was it first noticed?
- Does the hearing loss fluctuate?
- Is there a family history of hearing loss?
- Is there a history of noise exposure – occupational or recreational?

As soon as a patient enters the room, one can start to gauge their hearing: can they understand a normal conversational voice? Patients who might be overexaggerating their hearing loss (for example, because of compensation claims or because they do not want to go to school) may still automatically respond without being able to see the clinician's face. It is interesting how many young teenagers, seemingly with a profound hearing loss on pure tone audiometry, can still hear when you ask a question from behind them!

CLINICAL ASSESSMENTS

▌ 'Whisper test'

The whisper test provides a useful, approximate, assessment of hearing loss that can be performed in any quiet environment. The sensitivity of the test, to detect a speech-frequency hearing loss of greater than 30 dB, was 96% and the specificity 91% in one study.[1] Each ear is tested in turn, with masking of the non-test ear provided by repeatedly pressing its tragus to occlude the meatus. The patient is asked to repeat numbers or words that you speak at arm's length (about 60 cm) from the test ear (**Figure 3.1**). At this distance, the volume of a whispered voice is approximately 30–40 dB, a normal talking voice about 50–60 dB, and a very loud voice about 80 dB. This provides approximate thresholds only and does not help assess loss at individual frequencies, nor does it give any clue as to the type of hearing loss (i.e. whether it is conductive, sensorineural or mixed). Masking of the contralateral ear is very important, as it provides about 60 dB of masking and makes the test more reliable until very loud test levels are used (shouting). In the past, a Barany box was used to mask the non-test ear, but the masking noise is too loud and will interfere with results in the test ear (overmasking), so it is not to be recommended.

▌ Tuning fork tests

There are a variety of tuning fork tests, and they can be helpful in providing information about the type of hearing loss a patient may have, but are not used for assessing thresholds.

Rinne's test

Rinne was a German physician who described this test in 1855. Rinne's test assesses the difference in perception of air conduction compared with bone conduction, and is best performed using a 512 Hz tuning fork. The tuning fork is struck against a firm, but not hard, surface, such as one's elbow, to produce a pure tone. The fork is then held about 2 cm from the test ear, with the tines in line with the ear canal (**Figure 3.2A**). The patient is asked to listen to that sound, and then the base of the fork is pressed to the mastoid bone behind the pinna (**Figure 3.2B**). It is important that firm counterpressure is applied to the other side of the patient's head – the test is very unreliable without this. The patient is asked which sound

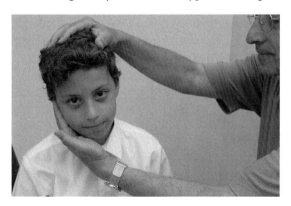

Figure 3.1. Photo of a whisper test in a clinic. Note the occlusion of the contralateral ear by digital pressure of the tragus.

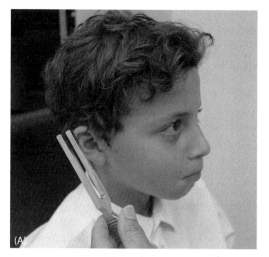

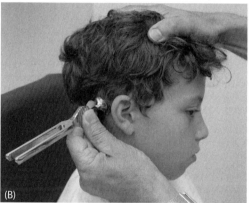

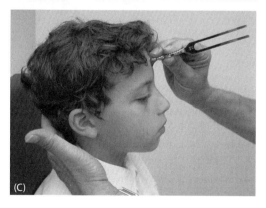

Figures 3.2A–C. Illustrations of tuning fork tests. (3.2A) Rinne's test: air conduction. Note the tines of the tuning fork are in line with the external auditory canal. (3.2B) Rinne's test: bone conduction. Note the counterpressure to the opposite side of the head. (3.2C) Weber's test. Note the counterpressure to the back of the head.

is louder: the first one (air conduction) or the second one (bone conduction). If air conduction is louder than bone conduction, this is a Rinne's positive result and occurs either in normal-hearing ears or ears with a sensorineural hearing loss. If bone conduction is louder than air conduction, this is a Rinne's negative result, and occurs if there is a conductive component to the hearing loss. Sometimes the patient cannot tell which is louder, and equivocal results can be interpreted as Rinne's negative – this improves the sensitivity of the test.[2] If a patient has a profound sensorineural hearing loss in one ear (a so-called 'dead ear'), a false-negative result will occur (bone conduction louder than air conduction), because the sound vibrations are hardly attenuated as they travel through the skull, and will stimulate the contralateral cochlea.

Rinne's test has a high specificity, but poor sensitivity.[2,3] If there is no conductive hearing loss present, Rinne's will be positive 96% of the time. The sensitivity of the test is poor when there is a small air–bone gap (about 45% with an air–bone gap of less than 10 dB), but improves as the degree of conductive hearing loss increases: with an air–bone gap of 30 dB or greater, Rinne's test is likely to be negative 90–95% of the time.

Weber's test

Weber, a German physiologist, described this phenomenon in 1834. In this test, the base of the tuning fork is placed on the patient's vertex or forehead, with counterpressure applied to the back of the head, and the patient is asked whether the sound is heard more loudly in one ear or whether it sounds central (**Figure 3.2C**). In patients with no, or symmetrical, hearing loss, the sound will be heard centrally, but in patients with an asymmetric sensorineural hearing loss, the sound will be heard in the better-hearing ear. In patients with a conductive hearing loss, the sound will be heard in the poorer hearing ear, assuming that the cochlear function is symmetrical. There are two theories as to why this might be. The first theory is known as the 'occlusion effect' whereby the vibrations from the tuning fork are conducted, with hardly any attenuation, to the deafer ear's cochlea, whereas the normal environmental sounds are not transmitted through its defective conduction pathway (external auditory canal, tympanic membrane, ossicular chain). Clinicians can experience this by performing the Weber's test on themselves, and then occluding one ear canal. The second theory is that in an ear with a normal conduction mechanism, sound vibrations from the tuning fork are conducted outwards from the bony skull to the external environment via this conduction route, and thus sound intensity is lost from that ear, whereas this does not happen to the same degree if there is a defective conducting mechanism.

There are little data in the literature regarding the sensitivity and specificity of Weber's test, but generally the results should be interpreted with care and used in conjunction with the history, examination and pure tone audiometry. One study showed Weber's lateralising to the wrong ear in up to 25% of children with a unilateral hearing loss[4], and it is even less sensitive in patients with bilateral hearing loss.

A summary of Rinne's and Weber's tuning fork test results is shown in **Table 3.1**.

Other tuning fork tests

Stenger's test is designed to detect patients with a non-organic hearing loss who claim that they cannot hear in one ear, but actually have good hearing. It relies on the premise that if the same tone is presented to each ear simultaneously, but at a different volume, one can only hear the louder tone. If the louder tone is presented to the apparently deaf side, the patient with a genuinely deaf ear will not hear that loud tone, but will hear the quieter tone in their normal ear, so will respond that they can hear a noise. Patients with a non-organic hearing loss will hear the louder sound in their 'deaf' ear, which will mask the quieter sound on their non-deaf side, so will say that they cannot hear anything. This is a difficult test to do with tuning forks, not least because the patient cannot be allowed to see that there are two tuning forks being presented, hence the reason it is usually performed with pure tones presented via headphones.

Table 3.1. Summary of Rinne's and Weber's results in various clinical scenarios.

	Right ear	Left ear
Bilateral normal hearing	Rinne's +ve	Rinne's +ve
	Weber's central	
RIGHT sensorineural hearing loss	Rinne's +ve	Rinne's +ve
	Weber's → LEFT	
RIGHT conductive hearing loss	Rinne's −ve	Rinne's +ve
	Weber's → RIGHT	
Bilateral conductive hearing loss (e.g. glue ear)	Rinne's −ve	Rinne's −ve
	Weber's probably central, could lateralise to ear with greater conductive hearing loss	
LEFT total sensorineural hearing loss ('dead' ear)	Rinne's +ve	Rinne's FALSE negative (heard by RIGHT cochlea)
	Weber's → RIGHT	

Bing's test is designed to test the fact that occlusion of the ear canal improves the perception of bone-conducted sounds unless there is a conductive hearing impairment. This is less reliable than Rinne's testing in detecting conductive hearing losses and, again, is now rarely used.

REFERENCES

1 Browning GG, Swan IRC, Chew KK (1989) Clinical role of informal tests of hearing *J Laryngol Otol* **103**:7–11.

2 Burkey JM, Lippy WH, Schuring AG *et al.* (1998) Clinical utility of the 512-Hz Rinne tuning fork test *Am J Otol* **19**:59–62.

3 Browning GG, Swan IRC (1988) Sensitivity and specificity of the Rinne tuning fork test *Brit Med J* **297**:1381–1382.

4 Capper JWR, Slack RWT, Maw AR (1987) Tuning fork tests in children (an evaluation of their usefulness) *J Laryngol Otol* **101**:780–783.

4

AUDIOLOGICAL ASSESSMENT OF HEARING

Richard D. Knight, Sarah Yorke-Smith & Victoria H. Parfect

Contents

INTRODUCTION

There are a variety of diagnostic audiological tests available. The choice of test depends on what we want to know about the patient's audiological status, and on what the patient is capable or willing to do.

This chapter outlines the main tests that are available, when the tests may be indicated, how they are interpreted and the clinical information that they can yield. Standard procedures are available for many of these tests at the British Society of Audiology website.[1]

PURE TONE AUDIOMETRY

Pure tone audiometry (PTA) is the investigation of choice when answering the question 'What is this patient's hearing like?' It will discriminate between a conductive and a sensorineural hearing loss and generate targets for hearing aid settings where applicable.

The patient is seated in a sound-proofed room and presented with pure tones through headphones (or earphones) and asked to respond, usually by pressing a button when a sound is heard (no matter how faintly). There is a standard test sequence for reducing the sound intensity presented and establishing the threshold level to within 5 dBHL. The test begins at 1 kHz and is then repeated at 250 Hz, 500 Hz, 2 KHz, 4 KHz and 8 KHz and, on occasion, intermediate frequencies. If a hearing loss is demonstrated, testing is continued with a bone conductor mounted on a headband. If the bone conduction hearing thresholds are better than air conduction, the difference represents a conductive hearing loss. Bone conduction thresholds that are worse than the normal hearing range (i.e. ≥20 dBHL) indicate a sensorineural hearing loss.

Masking is often required as part of the test, because in some situations sound presented to one ear may be detected by the other ear. The masking noise is filtered white noise centred on the frequency under test and is applied to the opposite ('non-test') ear. The following rules apply when masking is required:

Rule 1. Air conduction in one ear is better than the other by ≥40 dB.
Rule 2. Bone conduction is better than air conduction by ≥10 dB.
Rule 3. Rule 1 has not been applied but unmasked bone conduction is better than air conduction by ≥40 dB.

The value of 40 dB is applied as it is a conservative estimate of interaural attenuation (i.e. the amount by which the sound level is reduced when travelling through the head from one ear to the other) when sounds are presented through headphones. Note that the masking noise is always presented by air conduction. In rules 1 and 3 the test tone is presented via air conduction during masking, whereas in rule 2 the tone is presented by bone conduction. Masking ensures that the responses obtained are from the ear that is being tested, since applying the masking noise to the non-test ear prevents it from detecting sounds presented to the test ear.

The test is generally reliable, with repeated tests usually varying by not more than 5 dBHL. However, there are some situations in which misleading results can be obtained. Where the ear canals are tortuous or nearly occluded with wax, the application of headphones or earphones can result in a full occlusion, and hence an apparent conductive hearing loss. Sometimes, for a variety of external or internal reasons, the patient may display non-organic behaviour and demonstrate an exaggerated hearing loss. Also, the patient's hearing may be distorted such that they can detect a sound but cannot interpret it clearly, and so their day-to-day difficulty may be greater than the audiogram would suggest. This can occur for cochlear (e.g. in Ménière's disease) or retrocochlear reasons.

A blank audiogram is shown in **Figure 4.1**. Note that the horizontal axis of the audiogram

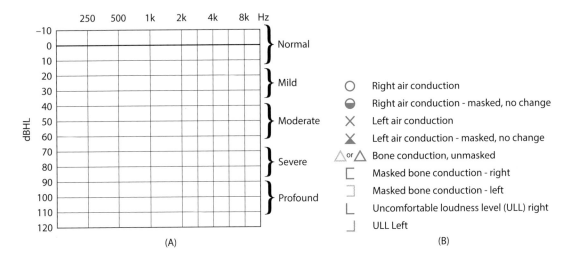

Figure 4.1. Audiogram, with current standard UK symbols.

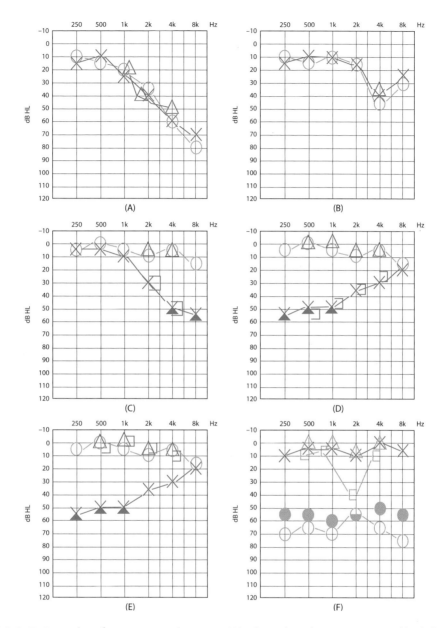

Figures 4.2A–F. Examples of pure tone audiograms. (A) Bilateral moderate symmetrical high frequency sensorineural hearing loss consistent with presbyacusis. (B) Bilateral mild symmetrical sensorineural hearing loss, notched at 4 kHz, typical of noise induced hearing loss. (C) Moderate left high frequency sensorineural hearing loss. An MRI scan is indicated to exclude a vestibular schwannoma. (D) Moderate 'reverse-slope' (low frequency) left sensorineural hearing loss (typical of early Ménière's disease). An MRI scan is also indicated. (E) A left conductive hearing loss (note normal left bone conduction). External and/or middle ear causes should be considered. (F) Right conductive hearing loss with 'Carhart notch' in bone conduction at 2 KHz. The notch is an artefact often seen in otosclerosis and there is unlikely to be a true sensorineural aspect to the hearing loss, since recovery of the bone conduction thresholds may be observed after a successful stapedectomy. The observed reduction in bone conduction thresholds may be attributable to the ossicular chain having a natural resonance frequency around 2 KHz, which is diminished when there is ossicular fixation.

displays ascending frequency from left to right and the vertical axis shows the sound presentation level with quiet levels (i.e. good hearing thresholds) towards the top and louder sound levels (i.e. poor hearing thresholds) towards the bottom. Descriptive terms of hearing levels are shown on the right, ranging from normal to profound.

Some examples of audiograms that may be obtained, along with the typical causes, are shown (**Figures 4.2A–F**).

TYMPANOMETRY

Tympanometry is a test of middle ear function that is simple and very quick to perform. It tests the admittance (or compliance) of the middle ear (that is, the flow of sound energy into the middle ear relative to that which is reflected). A soft probe tip is placed in the ear canal to achieve an air-tight seal. The probe plays a low frequency tone and sweeps across a range of air pressures in the ear canal while measuring the admittance (or compliance) of the eardrum. The patient does not need to respond but does need to sit still without swallowing or talking.

Tympanometry is useful for investigating the mobility and integrity of the eardrum. For example, the test can be used to obtain more information about a conductive hearing loss, equivocal bone conduction audiometry and audiograms, without bone conduction results (this sometimes occurs in young children when attention spans can be short, resulting in an incomplete audiometry test). It is also possible to determine whether there is a perforation in the eardrum, as the test result includes a value for the volume of air sealed in the ear canal by the tympanometry probe tip (an excessively large volume indicates a perforation, as the volume figure then includes the middle ear space). Some example tympanograms and typical causes are shown (**Figures 4.3A–E**), with normal values shown in **Table 4.1**. Note that in some centres the Jerger (1970) results classifications are used to report tympanometry results. These are shown in brackets in the figure caption, although this classification is no longer carried within the British standard for this test (British Society of Audiology Recommended Procedure Tympanometry June 2014).[2]

Contraindications for the test include excessive wax close to the entrance to the ear canal (this should be removed before the test), external ear infection or a history of recent middle ear surgery (the pressure changes involved in the test may damage the surgical repair).

Table 4.1. Normal ranges for adult tympanometry.

Parameter	Range
Middle ear pressure relative to atmospheric pressure	−50 to +50 daPa in adults, although down to −100 daPa or even lower may not be of clinical significance in young children
Compliance or admittance	0.3–1.6 cm³, although minor deviations from this range may not be of clinical significance
Ear canal volume	0.6–2.5 cm³ in adults, needs to be consistent with the observed ear canal size

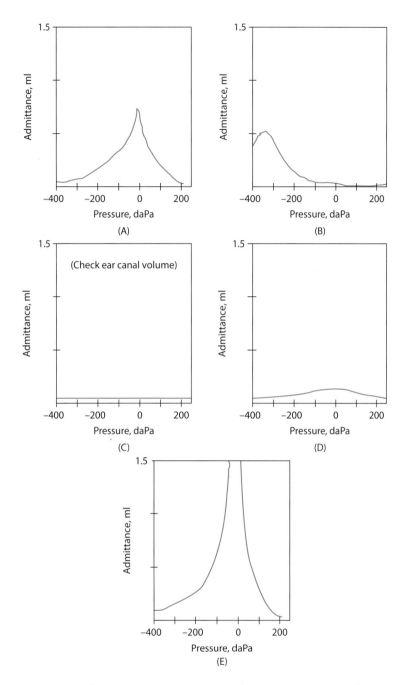

Figures 4.3A–E. Some example tympanograms. (A) Normal (type 'A'). (B) Reduced middle ear pressure, the eardrum may appear retracted (type 'C'). (C) A flat trace, can be due to a middle ear effusion (normal middle ear canal volume), wax occlusion (reduced ear canal volume) or an eardrum perforation (large ear canal volume) (type 'B'). (D) A low peak indicating low compliance. This may occur for example in cases of tympanosclerosis. It can also sometimes be seen in otosclerosis, although with low sensitivity and specificity.[2] (E) Hypercompliant tympanic membrane, found with an excessively flaccid eardrum or ossicular chain discontinuity (type 'Ad').

STAPEDIAL REFLEXES

Testing the stapedial reflexes is useful for investigating the auditory pathway as well as the descending branch of the facial nerve to the stapedius muscle. There are various theories regarding the purpose of the stapedial reflex:

- Protection of the cochlea from excessively loud sounds.
- Improving clarity of higher frequency hearing by reducing the upward spread of masking from the lower frequency components.
- The middle ear muscles may hold the ossicles in place and control rigidity.
- Optimisation of middle ear function for transmission of sound to the cochlea.

The stapedius muscle contracts as a reflex when a loud sound is presented. The neural pathway involves the ascending ipsilateral path to the brainstem and then bilaterally back to contract both stapedius muscles (**Figure 4.4**). The test can therefore be performed ipsilaterally (sound stimulus and recording in the same ear) or contralaterally (stimulus in the one ear and recording in the other ear). The test is performed by inserting a tympanometry tip into the ear, equalising air pressure across the eardrum, and then presenting a brief tone while looking for fluctuations in the measured eardrum admittance, caused by contraction of the stapedius muscle. The test is commonly performed at octave frequencies from 500 Hz to 4 kHz.

In normal subjects a response threshold may typically be around 85–95 dBHL. Although the test is not routinely performed, there are several instances in which it may be useful:

- To determine whether or not the stapes footplate is free in order to support the likely diagnosis of otosclerosis (in which case only ipsilateral responses for the opposite ear may be measureable, or it may be possible to measure a contralateral but not ipsilateral response when stimulating the affected side).

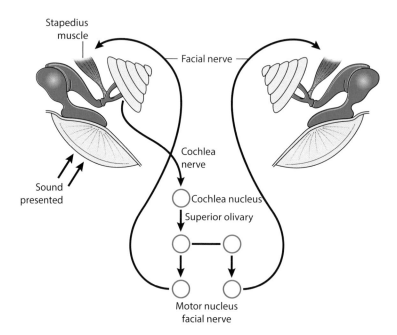

Figure 4.4. Diagramatic illustration of the pathways involved in the stapedial reflex.

- Investigation of the retrocochlear pathway to gain an insight into the site of the lesion (e.g. in cochlear nerve pathology it may be possible to stimulate the reflex contralaterally but not from the ipsilateral side).
- Investigation of possible non-organic hearing loss (if a response is seen to a stimulus and the patient denies hearing, a non-organic hearing loss is suggested).
- Investigation into facial nerve pathology (e.g. in Bell's palsy, in which case there may be no acoustic reflex seen on the affected side regardless of which side is stimulated).
- Determining whether a mild or moderate hearing loss is conductive or sensorineural (in sensorineural hearing loss there is little change in the stapedial reflex threshold, whereas in conductive hearing loss the reflex threshold changes by the full extent of the hearing loss).

Care should be exercised in interpreting contralateral results because, for example, a test playing a stimulus to the right ear and recording a response from the left may be considered to be either a right contralateral or a left contralateral recording depending on whether the side of test is being labelled by the stimulus or recording. This should always be made clear on the results table. Care should also be taken if performing this test on a subject reporting reduced loudness tolerance. Some example configurations of results that may be seen are shown in **Table 4.2**.

In the event of brainstem pathology, various configurations of results are possible including loss of contralateral responses, unilaterally absent responses or, in larger lesions, a 'full house' of absent responses. In the event of otosclerosis, result configurations seen in parts B or C may be seen depending on the extent of hearing loss.

A test that is related to stapedial reflexes is long-time-based tympanometry. In this test, air pressure is equalised across the eardrum and then the

Table 4.2. Some example configurations of results that may be seen.

A		Stimulus	
		Ipsilateral	**Contralateral**
Recording	Right	Present	Absent
	Left	Absent	Present
A: No response to stimulus on left side; left peripheral or vestibular nerve pathology.			

B		Stimulus	
		Ipsilateral	**Contralateral**
Recording	Right	Absent	Absent
	Left	Present	Present
B: No response measurable on right side regardless of which side is stimulated; right facial nerve pathology.			

C		Stimulus	
		Ipsilateral	**Contralateral**
Recording	Right	Absent	Absent
	Left	Present	Absent
C: No response to either stimulus or recording on the right side; right middle ear pathology. In mild cases the contralateral recordings may be recordable but with a raised threshold.			

compliance of the eardrum is monitored for an extended time, perhaps 10 or 15 seconds. This can be useful in patients with:

- Patulous Eustachian tube (measure with the patient breathing and then holding their breath and look for oscillations in compliance in association with breaths).

- Stapedius or tensor tympani muscle myoclonus (looking for bursts of fluctuations in compliance in association with bursts of reported myoclonus).
- Investigation of pulsatile tinnitus (if corresponding pulse-synchronous oscillations are seen, this may establish the mechanism of the tinnitus to be vascular).

SPEECH AUDIOMETRY

Speech audiometry is designed to assess the clarity/usefulness of a patient's hearing. Therefore, it may be of value in cases where the patient reports hearing difficulty in excess of what may be expected from the audiogram. There is no single standard format for speech audiometry and the speech material employed can range from simple phonemes (basic distinctive units of speech sounds) to single words or full sentences. When results are being interpreted it should be remembered that the real world environment differs significantly from this test environment, with additional background noise, competing foreground noise sources and non-auditory distractions. Nevertheless, speech audiometry does provide additional evidence of hearing clarity that may not be identified by pure tone audiometry.

One example of a common format of speech audiometry is to present pre-recorded lists of 10 consonant-vowel-consonant (CVC) words (the Arthur Boothroyd 'AB wordlists'). The patient is then asked to indicate what they have heard (after each single word – it is not a memory test!). This is usually done by asking the patient to repeat the word out loud, although writing it down is acceptable. The patient is scored on each phoneme in the word (i.e. 3 per word or 30 per word list). Additional lists of words are presented at different sound levels until a curve is generated.

A typical chart is shown in **Figure 4.5**. Although various factors can be reported from this chart, the main clinical interest focuses on the maximum score, the sound level at which this occurred, and

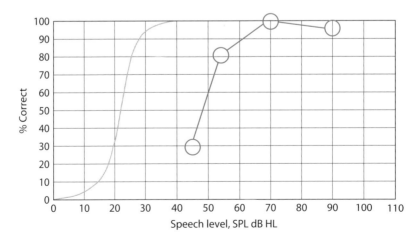

Figure 4.5. An example speech audiogram. In this case the result is typical of a mild hearing loss.

the presence or absence of any 'roll over' (deterioration of the score towards higher presentation levels), which can indicate retrocochlear pathology.

Speech audiometry can give a useful indication of distorted hearing and indicate the usefulness of remaining hearing, for example in patients with vestibular schwannomas or who are suffering from cochlear distortion of their hearing, as can occur in Ménière's disease. This assists with counselling the patient regarding the potential benefit from hearing aids. The test can also be useful in non-organic cases in which a better than expected result may be obtained or non-physiological patterns may be seen (e.g. always responding with one incorrect sound in the word or responding to alternate words).

OTOACOUSTIC EMISSIONS

Otoacoustic emissions are acoustic responses measured in the ear canal, normally following an acoustic stimulus. This response is a by-product of the normal activity of the OHCs of the cochlea. There are two main formats of this test available:

1 Transient evoked otoacoustic emission (TEOAE): a click stimulus is presented and a response is obtained between approximately 3 and 20 milliseconds afterwards. The response is separated from the stimulus by time.
2 Distortion product otoacoustic emission (DPOAE): a pair of tones is presented simultaneously (frequencies f_1 and f_2) and a response is measured simultaneously at a different frequency (frequency $2f_1-f_2$).

Successful recording of TEOAE requires near normal cochlear function and is the first-line test in newborn hearing screening, where automated TEOAE are performed. DPOAE can also be used for the same purpose but as a small response can be recorded in moderate hearing loss, more stringent minimum response level criteria are added when used as a screening tool. As DPOAE can be seen in the presence of greater hearing loss than TEOAE, and also may be recordable to higher frequencies, DPOAE is often the format employed as part of a diagnostic investigation and also for monitoring of cochlear function, for example in patients treated with ototoxic drugs.

Measurements are made by inserting an ear tip containing a loudspeaker and a microphone into the ear canal. The patient simply needs to sit still and quiet while the test is run. This may take between 20 seconds and a few minutes.

As OAE measurement requires sound to travel in and out through the middle ear, any middle ear losses are double-counted, so even the smallest of conductive hearing losses may abolish the OAE response. Other clinical uses for OAEs include:

● Investigating the status of peripheral function in known retrocochlear pathology.
● In patients with suspected non-organic hearing loss, the presence of OAEs can indicate a high likelihood of near-normal hearing.

AUDITORY BRAINSTEM RESPONSE

The auditory brainstem response (ABR) test may be useful in various contexts:

● In newborn hearing screening if they repeatedly fail OAE testing or where patients have a higher risk for hearing loss following admission to the SCBU (Special Care Birth Unit) or NICU (Neonatal Intensive Care Unit) at birth.
● To gain an estimate of hearing thresholds where an audiogram is not possible or is of doubtful reliability. This can occur in

non-organic hearing loss, where the patient does not understand what is required of them in performing an audiogram or where they are physically unable to provide a clear response to a sound.

- To investigate possible retrocochlear pathology, for example in patients who cannot undergo an MRI or to explore the impact of known retrocochlear pathology on the auditory pathway.

The ABR is an electrical measurement, via electrodes on the skin, of the first part of the auditory system up to the inferior colliculus. An auditory (or occasionally electrical) stimulus is presented to the ear. This classically takes the form of broad frequency range clicks (but can also be tonepips, which are more frequency specific) or other sounds such as 'chirps' (a specialised form of click intended to produce a sharper response waveform). A series of characteristic waves (labelled from I–V) arising from different parts of the early neural auditory pathway are recorded over the following few milliseconds (**Figure 4.6**). Repeated presentations of the sound allow averaging of the response and an associated improvement in the signal-to-noise ratio of the waveform.

A critical aspect of this test is that the patient must be relaxed, although ideally asleep in order to avoid electrical noise from muscle activity. This can usually be achieved in cooperative adults and in young babies, but older babies and young children often require sedation or a general anaesthetic.

The test can be subdivided into two categories depending on whether the goal is to measure a response 'threshold' or whether the goal is diagnostic (to investigate possible retrocochlear pathology). In both cases, the active electrode is placed on the mastoid, with reference electrodes on the forehead and, sometimes, the vertex or sternum.

For a diagnostic ABR, it is usual to measure at a single fairly high stimulus level (commonly 80 or 90 dB nHL) and the latencies of each wave are investigated closely. Excessive latency between waves is suggestive of pathology affecting either the cochlear nerve or brainstem, as is the absence of later waves (e.g. wave III or V) in the presence of the early waves.

A threshold ABR is measured at several stimulus levels with the aim of determining the minimum level at which wave V can be reliably recorded, most commonly performed to estimate hearing threshold in babies. As it is the latest and usually strongest wave, the main interest is in the presence or absence of wave V.

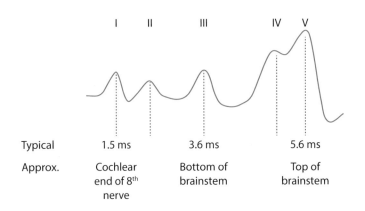

Figure 4.6. A typical diagnostic auditory brainstem response waveform.

VISUAL REINFORCEMENT AUDIOMETRY

Visual reinforcement audiometry (VRA) is a conditioned behavioural assessment employed widely across paediatric audiology to assess hearing levels in infants. VRA is applicable from 6 months of age when infants, following normal developmental milestones, are able to sit upright with support and have sufficient neck control to make head turns. It is used until 30 months of age, or older for children with developmental delay. VRA uses a visual reward to condition the infant head turn in response to sound stimuli (**Figure 4.7**). Good visual acuity is required, although modification of visual or tactile rewards is employed in cases of visual impairment. Interesting and varied visual reinforcers facilitate thorough ear and frequency specific results; examples include animated toys lit up behind smoked glass, flashing lights and computer animations. During testing the infant's attention is focused forward, using play distraction at a level that keeps the infant interested but not so engrossed to prevent turning to sound stimuli. In the initial conditioning phase of VRA, suprathreshold sound stimuli are delivered simultaneously with the visual reinforcer, the infant learning that turning to sound results in a visual reward. Sounds are then presented in the absence of visual reinforcement, with the visual reward only presented subsequently if the infant turns in response to the sound, strengthening conditioning and ensuring reward is only associated with audible sound presentation. The sound stimuli can then, as with PTA, be systematically presented in descending and ascending presentations, and in this way ear and frequency specific minimum response levels (MRLs) and hearing thresholds in infants can be assessed. The VRA paradigm allows air and bone conduction assessment via soundfield speakers, headphone, insert earphone and bone conduction presentation. Insert earphones/headphones are required to gain ear specific information, as soundfield presentation via speakers represents hearing from the 'better ear' with both ears working together.

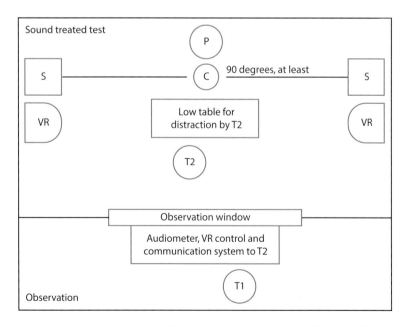

Figure 4.7. Schematic visual reinforcement audiometry room set-up. C, child on small chair or parent/carer's lap; P, parent/carer; S, speaker; VR, visual reinforcers; T1, tester (audiologist) controlling sound stimuli and VR timing; T2, controlling child's attention.

MRLs are different to PTA thresholds, since the infant's hearing levels may be better than the levels presented. VRA should be carried out by trained and experienced audiologists, aware of the potential pitfalls that affect the accuracy of this assessment; for example, false positives/negative responses from unintentional cues, loss of infant interest and inadequate distraction.

PLAY AUDIOMETRY

Play audiometry is an adapted form of PTA suitable for children aged from approximately 30 months to 6 years old. In PTA, adults are taught to respond to sounds by pressing a button. In play audiometry this response is exchanged by conditioning a child to perform a simple action response using play and toys. An example is to teach a child to put a wooden man in a toy boat every time they hear a sound; a variety of 'games' should be available to maintain attention and accuracy. Initially the 'game' is taught/demonstrated using supra-threshold stimuli with encouragement and reward when the child correctly links the sound to the response. If the child responds without a sound, this response must be 'undone' (e.g. removing the man from the boat) to prevent false-positive responses and inaccurate results. The 'games' must: elicit a response that is repeatable and not ambiguous; have enough responses to record multiple thresholds/ frequencies; and be interesting enough to maintain a child's attention but not be too engrossing. As with PTA testing, stimuli are delivered by an audiometer via insert earphones/headphones/bone conductor to obtain ear and frequency specific thresholds. Masking is possible depending on the ongoing accuracy of responses and attention of the child. An abbreviated PTA technique may be employed for the order of sound presentations and fewer thresholds may be acquired in comparison with adult PTA to ensure maximum accurate information within the time dictated by the child's attention. If the child is non-compliant or wary of headphones, initial testing can be carried out in the sound field (with a hand held warbler or speakers), referred to as 'performance audiometry'; this, as with soundfield VRA, reflects overall hearing and is not ear specific.

ELECTROCOCHLEOGRAPHY AND PROMONTORY STIMULATION

Tests within this category can be employed to provide a diagnostic test for Ménière's disease and to provide evidence of a functioning auditory nerve in cases of profound hearing loss. Recordings are made of the summating potential and/or the action potential. The summating potential is the response of hair cells as they move with the basilar membrane. The action potential is the response of the auditory nerves firing in response to depolarisation of the IHCs.

It is possible to record electrical responses from within the cochlea by positioning a recording needle electrode on the promontory of the middle ear. This is usually placed directly through the tympanic membrane.

▌ Electrocochleography

Electrocochleography (**Figures 4.8A–C**) classically involves presenting clicks and recording the summating potential and action potential from the cochlea. Using a 90 dB nHL click, a waveform such as that shown in **Figure 4.8A** is obtained. The primary use for this test is to support the diagnosis for Ménière's disease (the test has a fair specificity but

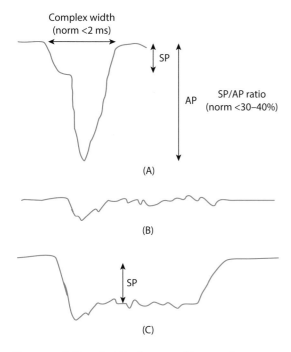

Complex width
(norm <2 ms)

SP

AP

SP/AP ratio
(norm <30–40%)

(A)

(B)

SP

(C)

Figures 4.8A–C. (A) Electrocochleography response to click stimulus. (B) Normal response to toneburst stimulation. (C) Response to toneburst stimulation suggestive of endolymphatic hydrops. SP, summating potential; AP, action potential.

poor sensitivity, quoted variously at between 20% and 65%[3]), and the parameters used are the amplitude ratio of the summating potential and action potential, with the normal range being typically below 30% or 40%. **Figures 4.8B and C** show waveforms that can be obtained from toneburst stimulation; this is an alternative recording paradigm whose results may have a stronger diagnostic value.

▌ Promontory stimulation

If an electrical stimulus is applied to the promontory, then it is possible to trigger the auditory nerve in the absence of IHCs and this can confirm the presence of a functioning cochlear nerve at the peripheral end. This can be useful when considering cochlear implantation in patients where it is not clear whether the cochlear nerve is working, such as in patients with neurofibromatosis type 2 and bilateral stable vestibular schwannomas with a profound hearing loss.

REFERENCES
1 http://www.thebsa.org.uk/resources/
2 Browning GG, Swan IR, Gatehouse S (1985) The doubtful value of tympanometry in the diagnosis of otosclerosis. *J Laryngol Otol* **(6):**545–547.
3 Hornibrooke J, Kalin C, Lin E *et al.* (2012) Transtympanic electrocochleography for the diagnosis of Ménière's disease. *Int J Otolaryngol* http://doi.org/10.1155/2012/852714.

5

IMAGING OF THE EAR

Steve Connor

Contents

INTRODUCTION

CT and MRI are the key modalities used to image patients with otological disorders. The high spatial resolution of CT is optimal for demonstration of the cortical bone and air spaces of the middle ear, mastoid and external auditory meatus (EAM) (**Figures 5.1A–N**), whereas the superior contrast resolution of MRI is ideal for imaging the inner ears, petrous apex and intracranial structures (**Figures 5.2A–H**). Cone beam CT (CBCT) is emerging as a 'low-dose' alternative to standard CT in certain clinical settings. This chapter will review the appropriate imaging in a range of clinical scenarios.

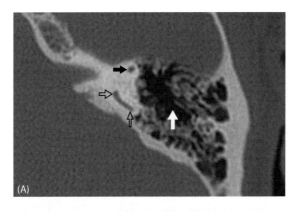

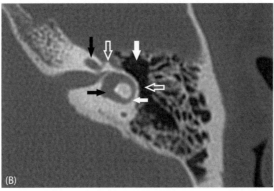

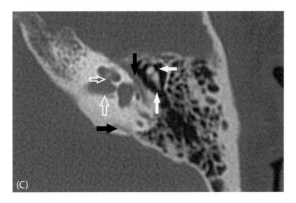

Figures 5.1A–N. CT images. Axial images from superior to inferior (5.1A–5.1G) and coronal images from anterior to posterior (5.1H–5.1N). (5.1A) Anterior limb superior semicircular canal (black arrow), common crus (horizontal open arrow), superior limb posterior semicircular canal (vertical open arrow) and mastoid antrum (white arrow). (5.1B) Vestibule (horizontal black arrow), superior segment basal turn of cochlea (vertical black arrow), aditus ad antrum (horizontal open arrow), geniculate ganglion/anterior genu of facial nerve canal (vertical open arrow), lateral semicircular canal (horizontal white arrow), epitympanum bordered anteriorly by tegmen tympani (vertical white arrow). (5.1C) Vestibular aqueduct (horizontal black arrow), tympanic portion of facial nerve canal (vertical black arrow), modiolus of cochlea, adjacent to cochlear aperture (horizontal open arrow), singular canal arising from dorsal internal auditory meatus (vertical open arrow), malleus head (horizontal white arrow), short process of incus projecting into incudal fossa (vertical white arrow). *(Continued)*

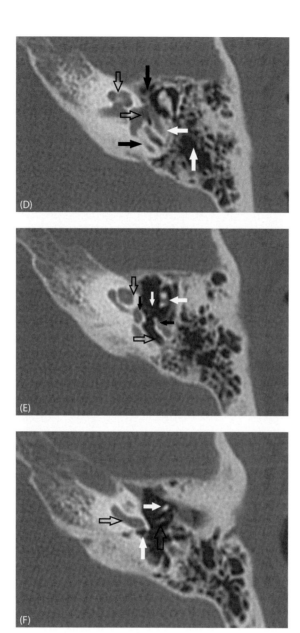

Figures 5.1A–N. (Continued) CT images. Axial images from superior to inferior (5.1A–5.1G) and coronal images from anterior to posterior (5.1H–5.1N). (5.1D) Posterior semicircular canal (horizontal black arrow), anterior epitympanic space in front of a bony septation-cog (vertical black arrow), oval window/stapes foot-plate (horizontal open arrow), notch and interscalar septa between middle and basal turn of cochlea (vertical open arrow), posterior genu of facial nerve canal (horizontal white arrow), posterior semicircular canal (vertical white arrow). (5.1E) Pyramid (horizontal black arrow), cochlear promontory (vertical black arrow), sinus tympani (horizontal open arrow), notch between middle and apical turn of cochlea (vertical open arrow), neck of malleus anteriorly with long process of incus posteriorly (horizontal white arrow), stapes (vertical white arrow). (5.1F) Inferior segment of cochlea basal turn with osseous spiral lamina just visible (horizontal open arrow), incudostapedial joint (vertical open arrow), handle of malleus (horizontal white arrow), round window niche (vertical white arrow). *(Continued)*

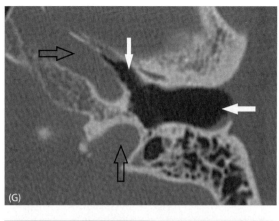

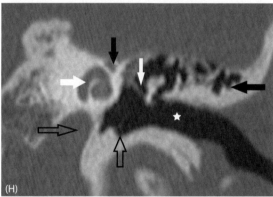

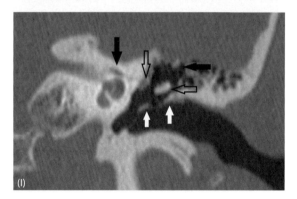

Figures 5.1A–N. (Continued) CT images. Axial images from superior to inferior (5.1A–5.1G) and coronal images from anterior to posterior (5.1H–5.1N). (5.1G) Horizontal portion of petrous carotid canal (horizontal open arrow), jugular bulb (vertical open arrow), external auditory meatus (horizontal white arrow), Eustachian tube (vertical white arrow). (5.1H) Tegmental air cells inferior to the tegmen mastoideum (horizontal black arrow), anterior genu of facial nerve canal (vertical black arrow), jugular fossa (horizontal open arrow), tympanic annulus adjacent to inferior pars tensa (vertical open arrow), basal turn of cochlea (horizontal white arrow), tensor tympani muscle attaching to neck of malleus (vertical white arrow), external auditory meatus (star). (5.1I) Tegmen tympani (horizontal black arrow), labyrinthine portion of facial nerve canal (vertical black arrow), body of incus (horizontal open arrow), tympanic portion of facial nerve canal (vertical open arrow), handle of malleus (short white arrow), scutum (long white arrow). *(Continued)*

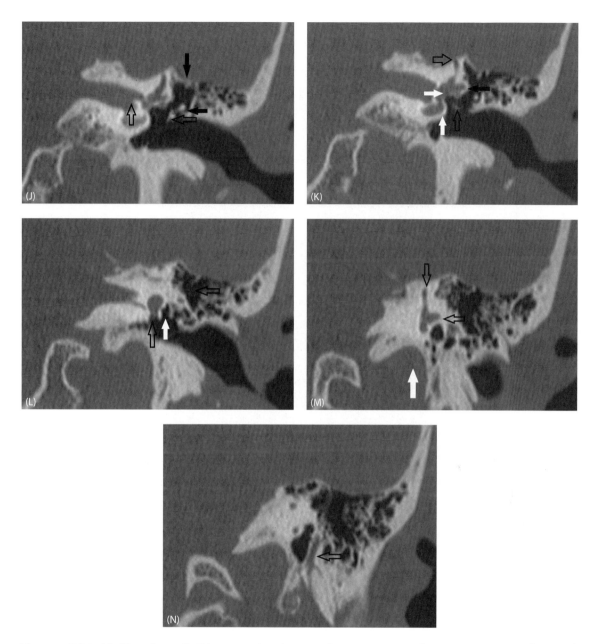

Figures 5.1A–N. (Continued) CT images. Axial images from superior to inferior (5.1A–5.1G) and coronal images from anterior to posterior (5.1H–5.1N). (5.1J) Short process of incus (horizontal black arrow), tegmen tympani (vertical black arrow), long process of incus (horizontal open arrow), crista falciformis at fundus of internal auditory meatus (vertical open arrow). (5.1K) Lateral semicircular canal (horizontal black arrow), a dehiscent superior semicircular canal (horizontal open arrow), incudostapedial joint (vertical open arrow), vestibule with adjacent oval window/stapes footplate (horizontal white arrow), cochlea promontory (vertical white arrow). (5.1L) Mastoid antrum (horizontal open arrow), round window (vertical open arrow), sinus tympani (vertical white arrow). (5.1M) Posterior limb of lateral semicircular canal (horizontal open arrow), posterior limb of superior semicircular canal (vertical open arrow), jugular fossa (vertical white arrow). (5.1N) Mastoid segment of facial nerve canal (vertical open arrow).

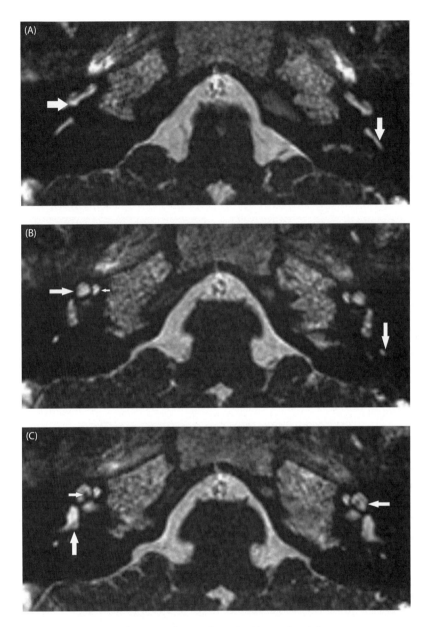

Figures 5.2A–H. MR images. Axial images from a heavily T2-weighted thin section sequence in which fluid returns high signal and which is designed to demonstrate the nerves within the internal auditory meatus and the inner ear structures. Figures 5.2A–5.2G are from inferior to superior; Figure 5.2H is a magnified image. (5.2A) Basal turn of cochlea (horizontal arrow) and inferior limb of posterior semicircular canal (vertical arrow). (5.B) Notch between middle and apical turns of cochlea (large horizontal arrow), descending segment of basal turn of cochlea (small horizontal arrow) and apex of posterior semicircular canal (vertical arrow). (5.2C) Notch between middle and basal turns of cochlea (large horizontal arrow), modiolus (small horizontal arrow) and vestibule at origin of common crus (vertical arrow). *(Continued)*

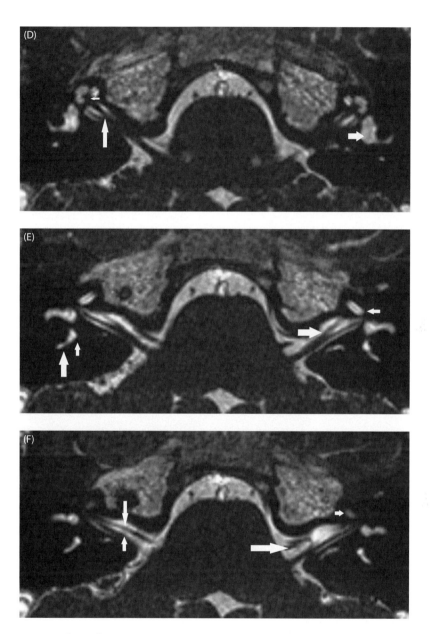

Figures 5.2A–H. (Continued) MR images. Axial images from a heavily T2-weighted thin section sequence in which fluid returns high signal and which is designed to demonstrate the nerves within the internal auditory meatus and the inner ear structures. Figures 5.2A–5.2G are from inferior to superior; Figure 5.2H is a magnified image. (5.2D) Vestibule (horizontal arrow), vestibulocochlear nerve with inferior vestibular (posterior)and cochlear nerve (anterior) divisions within the fundus of the internal auditory meatus (vertical arrow). (5.2E) Vestibulocochlear nerve with inferior vestibular (posterior) and cochlear nerve (anterior) divisions within the fundus of the internal auditory meatus (large horizontal arrow), superior segment of basal turn of cochlea (small horizontal arrow), superior limb of posterior semicircular canal (large vertical arrow) and common crus (small vertical arrow). (5.2F) Intrameatal vascular loop (large horizontal arrow), superior segment of basal turn of cochlea (small horizontal arrow), facial nerve (large vertical arrow) and vestibulocochlear nerve medially becoming superior vestibular nerve laterally (small vertical arrow). *(Continued)*

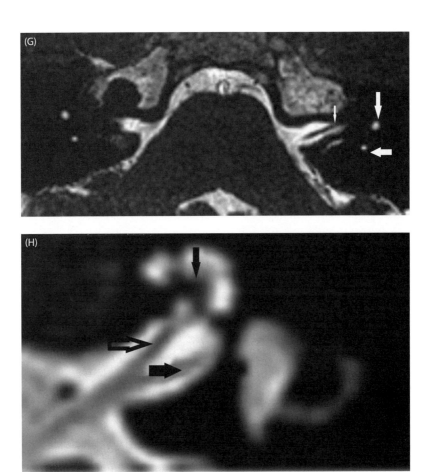

Figures 5.2A–H. (Continued) MR images. Axial images from a heavily T2-weighted thin section sequence in which fluid returns high signal and which is designed to demonstrate the nerves within the internal auditory meatus and the inner ear structures. Figures 5.2A–5.2G are from inferior to superior; Figure 5.2H is a magnified image. (5.2G) Posterior limb of superior semicircular canal (horizontal arrow), anterior limb of superior semicircular canal (large vertical arrow) and facial nerve at fundus of internal auditory meatus (small vertical arrow). (5.2H) The delineation of the cochlear nerve (open arrow), inferior vestibular nerve (black arrow) at the fundus of the internal auditory meatus. The internal architecture of the cochlea is shown with the interscalar septae radiating from the modiolus (vertical black arrow).

INFLAMMATORY DISEASE

Acute otitis media is a clinical diagnosis and does not require imaging. If there is evolution to 'clinical mastoiditis', then imaging is indicated to assess for coalescent mastoiditis, extracranial abscess and intracranial complications (e.g. sigmoid sinus thrombosis, cerebral abscess). CT with intravenous contrast is generally used in the emergency setting, while MRI plays a complementary role in demonstrating petrous apex and intracranial sepsis (**Figure 5.3**).

Otitis media with effusion may require imaging if it is persistent and unilateral. CT or MRI is then used to exclude a submucosal nasopharyngeal or deep facial mass as a cause of Eustachian tube obstruction.

Chronic suppurative otitis media (CSOM) may require radiological assessment, principally for the detection, preoperative planning and monitoring of cholesteatoma.[1] There are wide variations in the use of imaging in this clinical setting. While cholesteatoma is generally diagnosed at otoscopy, CT plays a role in clinically equivocal cases (**Figure 5.4**) or when otoscopy is not possible (e.g. external auditory meatus is obstructed). CT may also be helpful

for preoperative planning in order to delineate the surgical anatomy (e.g. extent of mastoid pneumatisation or anatomical variants), while CT and MRI may help define the extent of cholesteatoma (e.g. intralabyrinthine or intracranial extension). Finally, MRI is increasingly applied to the postoperative monitoring for recurrent cholesteatoma following combined approach tympanoplasty, and as an alternative to the traditional 'second look' surgery. MRI with non-echo planar diffusion-weighted imaging sequences is very effective for detecting recurrent cholesteatomas greater than 3 mm in size (**Figure 5.5**).

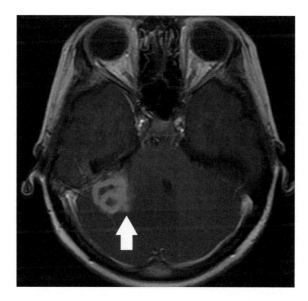

Figure 5.3. T1-weighted post-gadolinium axial MR image demonstrating a right cerebellar hemisphere enhancing abscess that was secondary to acute mastoiditis and that had spread through an eroded sigmoid plate.

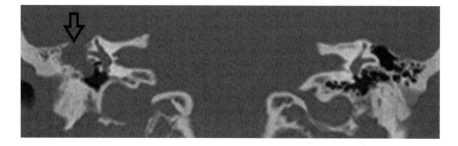

Figure 5.4. Coronal CT study showing non-dependent right middle ear soft tissue with an inferior convexity. Erosion of the tegmen tympani (arrow) and some attenuation of bone over the lateral semicircular canal is demonstrated (compare with the contralateral side). The features are highly suggestive of a cholesteatoma.

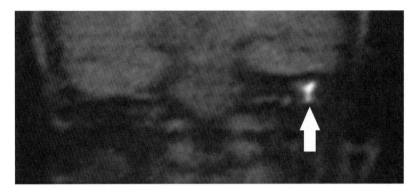

Figure 5.5. Coronal non-EPI diffusion-weighted MR image showing the increased signal returned by cholesteatoma (arrow).

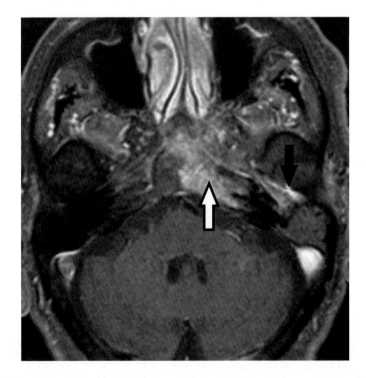

Figure 5.6. Axial T1-weighted fat saturated post-gadolinium MR image demonstrating the enhancing tissue within the central skull base and preclival region, secondary to necrotising otitis externa and secondary skull base osteomyelitis (open arrow). The source of the infection (i.e. external ear) is indicated by the tongue of enhancement within the left retrocondylar region (filled arrow).

Necrotising otitis externa should be imaged for diagnosis and to demonstrate its extent. While CT may demonstrate the early changes of tympanic bone erosion, MRI with gadolinium better shows the involvement of the subcranial soft tissues and the central skull base (**Figure 5.6**). Radioisotope studies are also sometimes used to monitor response to treatment.

CONDUCTIVE HEARING LOSS[2]

CT will be indicated in the setting of conductive hearing loss (CHL) when there is associated CSOM, congenital aural dysplasia, trauma or an otoscopically visible mass. The role of CT in the setting of CHL and normal otoscopy (with a clinical suspicion of otosclerosis) is more controversial. CT is >95% sensitive for the bony changes of otosclerosis (**Figure 5.7**), and some otologists find it useful in order to exclude alternative diagnoses, demonstrate variant anatomy and delineate the extent of otosclerosis for prognosis and treatment planning.

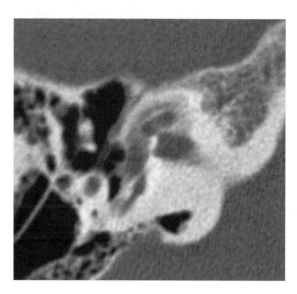

Figure 5.7. Axial CT image showing diffuse lucency within the perilabyrinthine structures, which indicates retrofenestral otosclerosis. Compare with the normal appearances of dense bone around the labyrinthine structures seen in the CT images in Figures 5.1A–N.

SENSORINEURAL HEARING LOSS[2]

Congenital sensorineural hearing loss (SNHL) is generally evaluated with MRI in order to diagnose macroscopic inner ear anomalies (**Figure 5.8**) (present in approximately 20% of cases), cochlear nerve integrity and brain abnormalities; however, a general anaesthetic may be required.

Acquired SNHL will require imaging investigation when it is asymmetric or unilateral. Imaging with thin section T2-weighted MRI sequences is primarily focused on the detection of cerebellopontine angle or internal auditory meatus mass lesions, such as vestibular schwannomas (**Figure 5.9**),

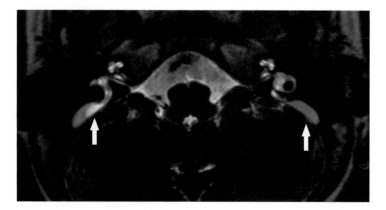

Figure 5.8. Axial heavily T2-weighted MR image demonstrating bilateral enlarged endolymphatic sacs and ducts (termed large vestibular aqueduct on CT imaging) in a patient with progressive sensorineural hearing loss (arrows).

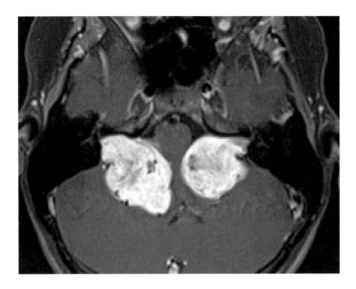

Figure 5.9. Axial T1-weighted post-gadolinium MR image showing bilateral enhancing cerebellopontine angle cistern and internal auditory meatus masses corresponding to vestibular schwannomas, in a patient with neurofibromatosis type 2. Note the marked brainstem compression.

which are present in 1–5% of such patients. In certain clinical settings (e.g. trauma, meningitis, immunosuppression), additional MRI sequences (e.g. T1-weighted and gadolinium enhanced) will be added and evaluation of the inner ear structures becomes more important.

AURAL AND EXTERNAL AUDITORY MEATUS DYSPLASIA

CT may be required to delineate bony anatomy as a precursor to bone conduction hearing aid or active middle ear implant insertion. CBCT may be appropriate, where available, in view of the higher risks of radiation exposure in children (**Figure 5.10**). Associated craniofacial anomalies and complications of EAM dysplasia (such as cholesteatoma) may also require documentation.

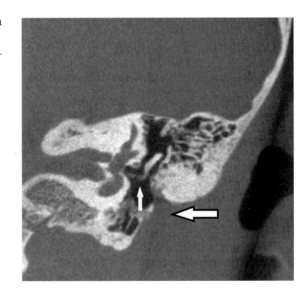

Figure 5.10. Coronal image from a CBCT study showing soft tissue atresia of the left external auditory meatus (horizontal arrow). The high resolution of the CBCT effectively demonstrates the incudo-stapedial joint (vertical arrow).

MIDDLE EAR MASS

A middle ear mass will most frequently corre-
spond to a glomus (jugulo) tympanicum. CT may
help distinguish a mass from vascular variants
(**Figure 5.11**), whereas CT and MRI (with gadolinium) are complementary in demonstrating the full
extent of the lesion.

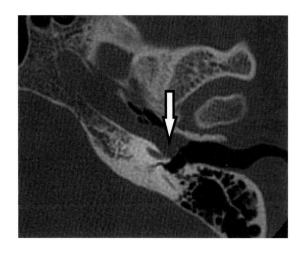

Figure 5.11. Axial CT image demonstrating extension of the left petrous carotid canal (arrow) into the
hypotympanum in a patient with an aberrant carotid
artery and a vascular middle ear mass.

OTALGIA[3]

Primary otalgia rarely requires CT or MRI for
diagnosis. Secondary (referred) otalgia may need
focused imaging if clinical features suggest an
alternative specific aetiology (e.g. temporomandibular joint, cervical spine, dentition). In the
absence of such clinical features, CT or MRI of the
whole neck may be performed to exclude an occult
tumour of the upper aerodigestive tract, particularly in a more elderly patient with relevant risk
factors.

TINNITUS[4]

Unilateral continuous tinnitus requires a similar
MRI protocol to that of asymmetric/unilateral
SNHL and is aimed at excluding a cerebellopontine angle or internal auditory meatus lesion.
Pulsatile tinnitus should be clearly identified on
an imaging request form, as this requires specific
imaging protocols (either with combined CT/CT
angiography/venography or MRI/MR angiography/
venography) in order to evaluate for potential
vascular tumours, anomalies, malformations and
stenoses.

FACIAL NERVE PALSY

MRI is indicated when the clinical course of a facial
nerve palsy is deemed to be atypical for a Bell's
palsy and there is clinical suspicion of a tumour
(or other lesion). It should be ensured that MRI is
performed with gadolinium, and that there is imaging coverage of the parotid gland and whole brain.

VERTIGO/DIZZINESS[5]

The majority of patients will be diagnosed with peripheral complaints, such as benign paroxysmal positional vertigo or Ménière's disease, and will not require imaging. MRI of the brain will be indicated if there are clinical features that indicate a central origin for the symptoms. This is usually combined with dedicated imaging of the internal auditory meatus, particularly if there are audiological features. In the emergency setting, CT of the brain may be used to demonstrate acute ischaemic or haemorrhagic lesions. Dedicated CT of the petrous bones also contributes in the setting of the post-traumatic or post-stapedectomy patient, in the context of CSOM and when semicircular canal dehiscence is suspected.

COCHLEAR IMPLANTATION

Pre-cochlear implant imaging is performed with MRI and/or CT. MRI is superior for demonstration of the cochlear nerve, the higher auditory pathways, inner ear anomalies and labyrinthine fibrosis/ossification, while CT is more beneficial for planning the surgical approach. Plain radiography and CBCT is selectively used in the peri- and post-implant setting in order to assess electrode position (**Figure 5.12**).

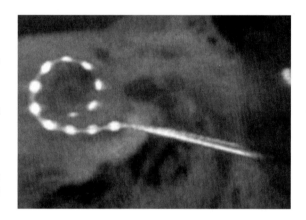

Figure 5.12. CBCT oblique coronal reformat demonstrates the position of the electrode contacts in a cochlear implant. CBCT results in less artefact from such metal implants compared with standard CT.

SYSTEMATIC ANALYSIS OF CT AND MRI

The review of an imaging examination should focus on the most clinically relevant anatomical features, but it is useful to develop a systematic review process. A potential approach is shown in **Tables 5.1 and 5.2**. The CT study may be reviewed from lateral to medial while the MRI study is reviewed from medial to lateral.

Table 5.1. Systematic review of petrous temporal bone computed tomography.

Review area	Specific features
Mastoid	• Pneumatisation • Size • Position of tegmen mastoideum • Course of facial nerve • Sigmoid sinus position • Post-surgical change
External auditory meatus	• Dysplasia • Defects/erosion • Soft tissue abnormality
Middle ear: • Epitympanum • Mesotympanum • Hypotympanum	• Aeration and morphology/density/distribution of any soft tissue abnormality • Ossicular integrity and continuity • Facial nerve dehiscence • Integrity of borders (floor, roof, scutum)
Middle ear anatomical variants	• Sinus tympani depth • Tympanic facial nerve protruding or medially situated • Jugular bulb dehiscent • Aberrant carotid canal
Oval window/fissula ante fenestram	• Thickness and size of oval window/stapes footplate • Otospongiotic plaques
Otic capsule	• Labyrinthine morphology/density/integrity • Peri-labyrinthine lucency
Petrous apex	• Erosive abnormality and aeration
Peri-auricular and subcranial soft tissue	• Change to 'soft tissue window'

Table 5.2. Systematic review of petrous temporal bone magnetic resonance imaging.

Review area	Specific features	Comment
Brain parenchyma		
Cerebellopontine angle cisterns and internal auditory meatus	• Mass lesions or neural irregularity • Presence and calibre of 7th and 8th cranial nerves	Beware 'normal variants' such as large cerebellar flocculus or vascular loops mimicking lesions
Inner ears	• Morphology • 'Fluid signal' present throughout on T2-W images • Peri-labyrinthine signal abnormality	Inner ear anomalies may be subtle (e.g. cochlear segmentation). Diffuse (e.g. fibrosis) or focal (e.g. intralabyrinthine tumour) signal abnormality may be present
Petro-mastoid and peri-auricular/subcranial regions		Analyse appropriate sequences, particularly in the setting of cholesteatoma, pulsatile tinnitus and complex skull base infection/tumour

REFERENCES

1 Baratk K, Huber AM, Stamppfli P *et al.* (2011) Neuroradiology of cholesteatomas. *Am J Neuroradiol* **32:**221–229.

2 Shah LM, Wiggins RH 3rd (2009) Imaging of hearing loss. *Neuroimaging Clin N Am* **19:**287–306.

3 Weissman JL (1997) A pain in the ear: the radiology of otalgia. *Am J Neuroradiol* **18:**1641–1651.

4 Weissman JL, Hirsch BE (2000) Imaging of tinnitus: a review. *Radiology* **216:**342–349.

5 Connor SE, Sriskandan N (2014) Imaging of dizziness. *Clin Radiol* **69:**111–122.

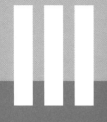

HEARING LOSS AND REHABILITATION

6

GENETICS OF HEARING IMPAIRMENT

Dirk Kunst

Contents

INTRODUCTION

The identification of genes that contribute to hearing and balance is helping to elucidate the molecular biology of the inner ear. In time, this research will lead to treatment strategies that prevent or stop the progression of hearing impairment: for example, by gene therapy. For this reason, it is important to keep abreast of new developments in the field of molecular biology of the inner ear.

Approximately 1 in 1,000 neonates are severely hearing impaired, with bilateral hearing thresholds of ≥80 dB. In at least half of these cases, the cause is inherited. The mode of inheritance can be autosomal recessive (70–80% of patients), autosomal dominant (20–30%) or X-linked (1–2%); mitochondrial inherited sensorineural hearing impairment (SNHI) has also been described. In approximately 70% of hereditary cases, no other stigmata related to SNHI can be recognized; these types of hearing impairment are classified as non-syndromic. The above mentioned data are mostly related to profound early childhood hearing impairment (prelingual phase). However, in the majority of patients with autosomal dominantly inherited hearing impairment, the age of onset is usually after early childhood (post-lingual phase). The prevalence of post-lingual SNHI in western Europe, with an average hearing threshold of >25 dB, is approximately 1% in young adults, about 10% up to the age of 60 years and almost 50% at 80 years. The degree to which hereditary causes contribute to hereditary post-lingual hearing impairment, and the prevalence of the different modes of inheritance, are unknown. Age-related hearing impairment is considered to be multifactorial, and is the result of both genetic and environmental factors.[1,2]

GENETIC DESCRIPTION OF HEARING IMPAIRMENT

The disease genes causing SNHI are expressed throughout the whole cochlea. The pathomechanisms of hearing impairment depend on the mutated gene and, therefore, on the function of the encoded protein in the inner ear. In addition, the type of mutation can play a role in terms of dominant and recessive mutations.

The locus on the chromosome that harbours a gene involved in non-syndromic autosomal dominant hearing impairment is specified by the prefix 'DFNA'. Non-syndromic autosomal recessive hearing impairment carries the prefix 'DFNB', while X-linked forms of non-syndromic hearing impairment are prefixed by 'DFNX'. About 64 DFNA, 101 DFNB and five DFNX loci are known. Many more loci are likely to be identified in the future. Approximately 30 genes for autosomal dominant, 55 genes for autosomal recessive and three for X-linked hearing impairment have been identified. There are more than 400 syndromes with hearing impairment as a feature and in many of these the associated gene has been identified. Much of these data are available via the Hereditary Hearing Loss website (http://hereditary-hearingloss.org).

GENETIC TESTING

Multiple technologies are available to identify the genetic defect underlying a clinically diagnosed hereditary hearing impairment. For example, linkage analysis can be used to confirm the inheritance of a disease allele in affected family members. Moreover, selected gene tests can confirm a genetic mutation as a cause of hearing impairment in an individual or family. Next generation sequencing techniques can be used to sequence a large panel of genes or the complete exome (whole exome sequencing) in a single experiment. Although whole exome sequencing has only recently been introduced into clinical practice, it is more efficient and cheaper than consecutive single gene sequencing.

CLINICAL DESCRIPTION OF HEARING IMPAIRMENT

In order to give an adequate clinical description of hearing impairment, several characteristics should be taken into account. These include age of onset, rate of progression, audiogram shape and severity. A tool to characterise different types of hearing impairment, based on pure tone audiograms, is the age-related typical audiogram (ARTA) method. This type of audio profiling reveals a comprehensive phenotype presentation in hearing impairment. If the genotype in a family is known, the corresponding ARTA can be used for counselling purposes. An ARTA can also help in predicting the gene involved in a specific family with hearing impairment.[3] Furthermore, it can be used to compare different types of hearing impairment in relation to the genotype. The construction of an ARTA from regression analysis of age-related pure tone threshold data has been described.[4,5] ARTAs belonging to different characteristic DFNA types are displayed in **Figures 6.1A–D**. An online tool for audio profiling of autosomal dominant hearing impairment, called Audiogene, is available at the webpage of the University of Iowa (http://audiogene.eng.uiowa.edu/).

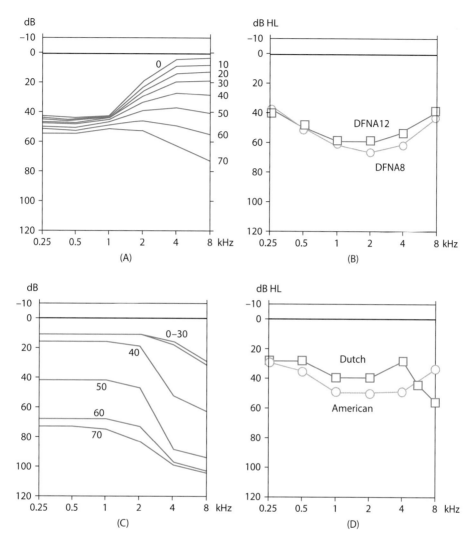

Figures 6.1A–D. (6.1A) Mean ARTA based on an American family and Dutch DFNA6/14 family. The gene involved is the *WFS1* gene. A low frequency sensorineural hearing impairment (SNHI) (40–50 dB) with no or mild progression is usually found. The numbers on the right of this figure represent the approximate age where the level of hearing loss is likely to be observed. (6.1B) Mean audiogram of DFNA8/12 family. Mutations in the *TECTA* gene cause a SNHI in which the mid-frequencies are most severely affected. Hearing may be stable over time. However, other mutations are known to cause progressive SNHI where the high frequencies are most affected. (6.1C) ARTA of a DFNA9 family. Mutations in the *COCH* gene cause a midlife onset SNHI with vestibular involvement. The SNHI, which might be asymmetrical, often progresses to profound impairment, for which cochlear implantation may be indicated. The numbers on the right of this figure represent the approximate age where the level of hearing loss is likely to be observed. (6.1D) Mean audiogram of two DFNA13 families. Mutations in the *COL11A2* gene usually cause a SNHI most pronounced at the mid frequencies. Only minor progression is usually seen.

RESULTS OF COCHLEAR IMPLANTATION

The results of cochlear implantation are excellent in patients with both syndromic and non-syndromic genetic hearing impairment associated with profound hearing loss. For example, in patients with Usher syndrome type I, the results are comparable with those obtained in other pre-lingual deaf patients. As with all cochlear implants, the outcome for the patient depends on confounding factors such as age at implantation and duration of deafness.

CONCLUSION

In recent years much progress has been made in the field of otogenetics. Many genes causing disease have been discovered and the corresponding phenotypes have been described. New diagnostic tests such as whole exome sequencing speed up developments even further. Otogenetics will become more important in daily clinical practice, facilitating the diagnostic process for the hearing impaired patient and making accurate counselling of prognosis possible.

REFERENCES

1 Fortnum HM, Summerfield AQ, Marshall DH *et al.* (2001) Prevalence of permanent childhood hearing impairment in the United Kingdom and implications for universal neonatal hearing screening: questionnaire based ascertainment study. *Brit Med J* **323(7312):**536–540.

2 Morton NE (1991) Genetic epidemiology of hearing impairment. *Ann N Y Acad Sci* **630:**16–31.

3 Bischoff AM, Luijendijk MW, Huygen PL *et al.* (2004) A novel mutation identified in the DFNA5 gene in a Dutch family: a clinical and genetic evaluation. *Audiol Neurotol* **9(1):**34–46.

4 Huygen PLM, Pennings RJE, Cremers CWRJ (2003) Characterizing and distinguishing progressive phenotypes in nonsyndromic autosomal dominant hearing impairment. *Audiol Med* **1:**37–46.

5 de Heer AM, Schraders M, Oostrik J *et al.* (2011) Audioprofile-directed successful mutation analysis in a DFNA2/KCNQ4 (p.Leu274His) family. *Ann Otol Rhinol Laryngol* **120(4):**243–248.

7

EXTERNAL EAR

Nick Saunders

Contents

PINNA ABNORMALITIES

Either one pinna or both may be congenitally small (microtia) or absent (anotia). This can be graded as grade 1 (pinna abnormal but recognisable), grade 2 (pinna abnormal, parts not recognisable; **Figure 7.1**), grade 3 (small auricular tag only) or grade 4 (anotia). Microtia is often associated with abnormalities of the ear canal and middle ear, and may be isolated or part of a syndrome such as Treacher Collins. Management ranges from hearing tests and simple reassurance to complex prosthetic or plastic surgical correction.

Prominent or otherwise misshapen ears may require surgical correction, generally just before school entry, but increasingly, techniques of early neonatal splintage are gaining acceptance and providing good results.

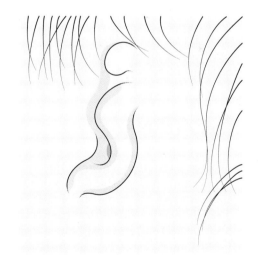

Figure 7.1. Microtia.

Trauma to the pinna may result in a haematoma, which if left untreated may result in a significant long-term cosmetic deformity ('cauliflower ear'). Perichondritis may also produce a similar outcome, as the elastic cartilage of the pinna derives its blood supply from the tightly adherent overlying perichondrium. If separated, the cartilage may undergonecrosis and fibrosis.

WAX

The ear canal is lined by skin and, as elsewhere in the body, there is constant turnover, with shedding of the superficial layer of squamous epithelium. However, desquamation of the skin of the tympanic membrane and ear canal occurs in an oblique fashion. This results in formation of an 'escalator mechanism' whereby keratin migrates laterally and, within the cartilaginous portion of the canal, mixes with various glandular secretions to produce wax (cerumen).

Many patients still use cotton buds to clean their ears. This should be actively discouraged as it often results in wax impaction and may traumatise the canal. The bony portion of the ear canal is bound to the underlying bone and is easily damaged.

FOREIGN BODIES

A variety of foreign bodies may be inserted into the ear canal. In children, beads, stones or other small items from toys or household goods may end up lodged in the canal. In adults, the tips of cotton buds or parts of hearing aids may become detached.

Unless there is resulting infection or significant trauma, removal is not an emergency, and can be carried out within a few days. Batteries are an exception, as they may start to leak and can be very corrosive; they should therefore be removed as soon as possible.

Removal of a foreign body is best done by someone with suitable skills and equipment, particularly in children, when the first attempt is most likely to be successful. If this fails, general anaesthesia may be required.

OTITIS EXTERNA

Otitis externa is a relatively common infection of the ear canal skin. Predisposing factors include skin conditions such as eczema or psoriasis, narrow ear canals, hearing aid use, trauma (including cotton bud use) and water exposure – hence the name 'swimmer's ear'. Common causative organisms are *Pseudomonas* species, other gram-negative organisms, *Staphylococcus aureus* and streptococci.

Otitis externa generally presents with pain and discharge. On examination, the skin of the ear canal is swollen and the tympanic membrane is often obscured by a combination of swelling and debris. Aural toilet (microsuction) may be required to remove this debris in order to allow effective treatment, which is generally with topical antibiotic drops or sprays; these often include a topical steroid. Occasionally, the causative organism may be fungal, in which case hyphae and spores are sometimes visible in the ear canal. In this situation it may be necessary to combine meticulous aural toilet with a course of antifungal drops lasting up to 4 weeks, as the drops are only active against growing fungi and not their spores. During treatment of the infection it is important that the patient takes precautions to keep water out of the ear when showering, bathing or swimming.

After resolution of otitis externa it is important to check the health of the tympanic membrane, as many cases of recurrent otitis externa are in fact secondary to recurrent discharge from a perforation or cholesteatoma.

Very rarely, recurrent infections may progress to chronic stenosing otitis externa. Chronic inflammation and circumferential scarring occur, with resulting stenosis of the canal that may then lead to an acquired atresia (blind ending canal). If this occurs, the infections usually stop but hearing may be significantly impaired due to the resulting conductive loss. Surgical correction is possible but not straightforward, and surgery should not be attempted while infections are still occurring.

SKULL BASE OSTEOMYELITIS (MALIGNANT OTITIS EXTERNA)

Skull base osteomyelitis is also called malignant otitis externa, a reflection of its potentially poor prognosis rather than any neoplastic process. It generally starts with a simple otitis externa and the causative organism is usually *Pseudomonas aeruginosa*. It almost exclusively affects patients with diabetes or another cause of immunosuppression, and should be suspected in any such patient in whom the infection proves difficult to control or if severe otalgia persists despite apparent clinical resolution of infection. Weakness of the lower cranial nerves often occurs, particularly the facial nerve. Treatment is best planned jointly with a microbiologist and usually requires a prolonged course of antibiotics, often initially intravenous for around 6 weeks followed by oral for several months. MRI is usually the best imaging modality, although resolution on imaging generally lags behind clinical resolution. A biopsy of external ear canal granulation tissue should be taken in order to exclude a squamous cell carcinoma, which may present with a similar clinical picture.

TUMOURS

True malignancy of the ear canal is, fortunately, rare. Squamous carcinoma may occur, particularly in patients with a long history of recurrent otorrhoea. Any patient with persistent ottorhoea and granulations in the ear canal should have a biopsy to exclude malignancy. Patients should be staged with MRI of the head to assess invasion of the dura or sigmoid sinus, as well as CT of the neck and chest to assess for metastatic spread.

Treatment is with radical surgery and radiotherapy, although the prognosis remains relatively poor.

Much more commonly, tumours may present on the skin of the pinna. Basal cell carcinomas, squamous carcinomas or melanomas may occur. Cartilage invasion is common and must be taken into account when planning excision.

OSTEOMAS/EXOSTOSES

Smooth, rounded bony lumps may occur in the ear canal. A solitary lump is usually an osteoma, which is a true benign bony neoplasm. Osteomata are rare.

Multiple lumps are almost always exostoses (**Figure 7.2**). These represent hypertosis rather than neoplasia and are generally found in the ears of patients with a history of immersion watersports (e.g. swimming, surfing), particularly in cold water. They are often asymptomatic and found incidentally, but may present with recurrent wax impaction or otitis externa. They are only very rarely themselves a cause of hearing loss. Most are managed conservatively, but if symptomatic they may be removed surgically.

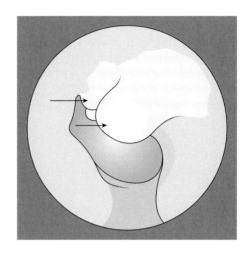

Figure 7.2. Exostoses of the external ear canal (arrows).

KERATOSIS OBTURANS AND EAR CANAL CHOLESTEATOMA

Keratosis obturans represents a failure of epithelial migration and presents with severe recurrent wax impaction, sometimes with expansion of the bony canal. The wax plug often has a characteristic lamellated structure. Treatment is with regular aural toilet.

In ear canal cholesteatoma, there is a focal ingrowth of squamous epithelium into the bony canal, usually the floor, often associated with an area of exposed bone. There may be significant pain and occasional discharge. Surgical treatment is usually required.

8 EUSTACHIAN TUBE DYSFUNCTION

Holger H. Sudhoff

Contents

INTRODUCTION

The Eustachian tube (ET) is a complex organ consisting of a dynamic, mucosal lined canal with its mucosa, cartilage, surrounding soft tissue, peritubal muscles, superior bony support and the sphenoid sulcus (**Figure 8.1**). The functions of the ET are pressure equalisation and ventilation

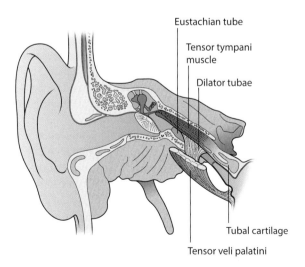

Eustachian tube
Tensor tympani muscle
Dilator tubae
Tubal cartilage
Tensor veli palatini

Figure 8.1. Temporal bone drawing of the cartilaginous and bony portion of the Eustachian tube and middle ear spaces including the major Eustachian tube muscles.

of the middle ear, mucociliary clearance of secretions and protection of the middle ear from sounds and from pathogens and secretions in the nasopharynx. Despite the improved knowledge of ET function, significant uncertainties remain. Our understanding of the anatomy and physiology of the ET still continues to evolve. The ET functions as a pressure-equalising valve for the middle ear, which is normally filled with gas. When functioning normally, the ET opens for a fraction of a second during swallowing or yawning. It allows air into the middle ear to replace air absorbed by the middle ear mucosa and to equalise pressure. Recently, it was shown that the ET may have a sequential peristaltic-like mechanism. ET dysfunction (ETD) is estimated to be present in about 1% of the general population. Almost 40 % of all children up to the age of 10 develop temporary ETD.

EUSTACHIAN TUBE DYSFUNCTION

ETD is still a poorly defined condition. It can either be acute or chronic. Acute ETD can occur during nasal congestion due to, for example, the common cold or allergic rhinitis, and is transient. ETD lasting longer than three consecutive months has to be considered chronic. Chronic ETD can be due to obstruction or to a patulous ET. ETD may lead to clinical symptoms such as aural fullness, impaired pressure equilibration, hearing loss and autophony. Because the most common cause of obstructive dysfunction is mucosal inflammation within the cartilaginous ET, patients should be questioned about inflammatory processes such as allergic rhinitis, chronic rhinosinusitis, laryngopharyngeal reflux and smoke exposure. Paediatric ETD may be caused by adenoidal hypertrophy and mucosal swelling due to upper respiratory tract infections. Predisposing factors for ETD include cleft palate, granulomatous diseases, cystic fibrosis, Sampter's triad or Kartagener's syndrome. It is important to distinguish ETD from other causes of aural fullness such as a patulous ET, temporomandibular joint disorders, superior semicircular canal dehiscence syndrome, Ménière's disease and increased intracranial pressure. The precise distinction between both forms of ETD – obstructive and patulous – is crucial. A patulous ET can be best diagnosed through a well-structured examination including patient history, physical examination with thorough observation of movements of the tympanic membrane, and tympanometry with reflex decay.

▌ Assessment

A large variety of methods have been employed to assess ET function, with more than 40 tests described in the literature. However, no single test is able to give detailed insights into all aspects of ET physiology and pathology. Otoscopy, endosocopy, Politzer test, Valsalva manoeuvre and Toynbee manoeuvre provide preliminary information. Manometric testing such as tympanometry and reflex decay tympanometry are in widespread clinical use. The nine-step inflation/deflation test, modified inflation/deflation test, forced response test and tubomanometry (TMM) have some additional value. TMM is a valuable tool to measure the opening of the ET tube and the transportation of gas into the middle ear by applying pressure changes in the nasopharynx and measuring the pressure in the external ear canal (EAC). Sonotubometry applies sound via a probe in the nose and records sound in the EAC during swallowing. Imaging using CT, cone beam CT and MRI are employed to access anatomical and functional deficiencies as well as to rule out pathology in the nasopharynx or superior canal dehiscence syndrome. Recent developments include a patient-rated ETD questionnaire (ETDQ-7) and an ET score (ETS7) that combine subjective and objective outcome measures. Despite extensive research, evidence guiding assessment and treatment of ETD patients is poor.

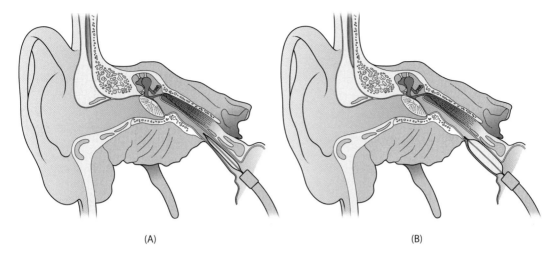

(A)   (B)

Figures 8.2A, B. Balloon dilatation tuboplasty of the cartilaginous portion of the Eustachian tube with a positioned catheter (A) and an inflated catheter at 10 bars for 2 minutes (B).

■ Treatment

Medical management of ETD should be directed at the underlying cause. Currently, there is little evidence of any efficient medical therapies for ETD. Pharmacological interventions include topical nasal steroids, antihistamines and decongestants. Various medical and surgical interventions are available for chronic obstructive ETD in a research setting including balloon Eustachian tuboplasty (BET) and laser or microdebrider tuboplasty (**Figures 8.2A, B**). Although studies are small, there is emerging work with encouraging but preliminary results. Recent treatment options, including BET and patulous ET surgery, may be offered to selected patients. Patients with patulous ETD may benefit from ET reconstruction with cartilage or injection of fat or debulking implants.

FURTHER READING

Bluestone CD, Klein JO (1996) Otitis media, atelectasis, and Eustachian tube dysfunction. In: *Pediatric Otolaryngology*, 3rd edn. (eds. CD Bluestone, SE Stool, MA Kenna) WB Saunders, Philadelphia.

Ockermann T, Reineke U, Upile T *et al.* (2010) A clinical study: balloon dilatation Eustachian tuboplasty (BET). *Laryngoscope* **120**:1411–1416.

Schröder S, Lehmann M, Sauzet O *et al.* (2015) A novel diagnostic tool for chronic obstructive Eustachian tube dysfunction: the Eustachian tube score. *Laryngoscope* **125**:703–708.

Seibert JW, Danner CJ (2006) Eustachian tube function and the middle ear. *Otolaryngol Clin North Am* **39**:1221–1235.

Sudhoff H (2013) *Eustachian Tube Dysfunction*. Uni-Med Verlag, Bremen, London, Boston.

ACKNOWLEDGEMENTS

Dr. Stefanie Schröder, Dr. Jörg Ebmeyer, Dr. Ulf Reineke, Martin Lehmann, Dr. Thorsten Ockermann, Dr. Dirk Korbmacher and Dr. Tarek Abdel-Aziz.

9 ACUTE OTITIS MEDIA AND OTITIS MEDIA WITH EFFUSION

Mahmood F. Bhutta

Contents

INTRODUCTION

Otitis media (OM) describes inflammation of the middle ear cleft (Eustachian tube [ET], tympanic cavity and mastoid air cells). In the developed world, acute otitis media (AOM) and otitis media with effusion (OME) are the most common forms of OM, and are highly prevalent diseases in infancy and early childhood.

ACUTE OTITIS MEDIA

AOM occurs due to ascent of resident bacteria from the nasopharynx up the ET into the middle ear space, leading to a purulent middle ear effusion. It is usually preceded by a viral upper respiratory tract infection, and the most common bacteria found in the middle ear are *Streptococcus pneumoniae*, non-typeable *Haemophilus influenzae* and *Moraxellla cattarhalis*.

AOM is the most common bacterial infection in childhood, affecting two-thirds of two-year-old children each year in the developed world. AOM is rare in older children and adults. Some children suffer recurrent AOM (rAOM), defined as ≥3 episodes of AOM in 6 months or ≥4 episodes in 12 months. If rAOM is associated with other recurrent mucosal infections, primary immunodeficiency should be excluded.

The aetiology of AOM is complex, and relates to exposure of an individual to new virulent strains of bacteria as well as individual susceptibility factors such as host genetics. Recognised risk factors in children are care in a nursery environment, having a sibling at home, household smoking and family history. In infants, breastfeeding offers some protection. Atopy is not a risk factor. Some texts suggest anatomical or functional variation in the ET is a risk factor, but there is little evidence to substantiate this claim.

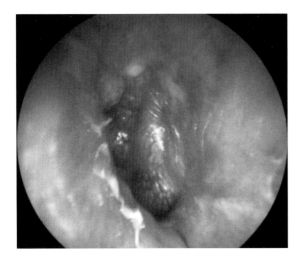

Figure 9.1. Otoscopic view of severe acute otitis media. The tympanic membrane is erythematous and bulging, with surrounding hyperaemia of the external auditory canal. (Courtesy David Pothier)

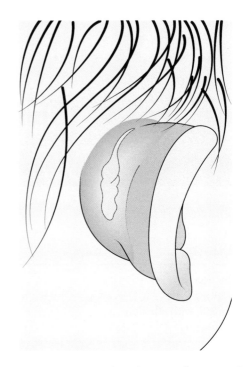

Figure 9.2. In 'mastoiditis' there is infection and erosion of the mastoid bone leading to a subperiosteal abscess behind the pinna.

AOM typically causes fever, malaise and unilateral otalgia. However, children under the age of two may not localise pain to the ear. Otoscopy classically shows erythema of the tympanic membrane (TM), with a purulent effusion and sometimes a bulging drum (**Figure 9.1**), although all these features are not necessarily present. In later stages the TM may perforate, resulting in otorrhoea of mucopus.

Treatment of AOM is usually symptomatic, as the disease typically starts to resolve 48–72 hours after onset. Analgesia should be prescribed. Antibiotics are not indicated in most cases because there is little benefit and a risk of side-effects such as diarrhoea and antibiotic resistance. Antibiotics (e.g. amoxicillin) may be considered in prolonged or severe cases: children aged under two with bilateral AOM, children with a fever >39°C or children in severe pain. Antihistamines, nasal decongestants and homeopathic treatments are not beneficial. Topical antibiotics should be considered if the TM has perforated.

Strategies for preventing rAOM include a 6-week course of low-dose antibiotics or insertion of grommets (ventilation tubes).

Serious complications of AOM are rare, but include mastoiditis, sigmoid sinus thrombosis, facial palsy, meningitis, temporal lobe abscess and Gradenigo syndrome (**Table 9.1**). 'Acute mastoiditis' describes when infection has spread through the lateral cortex of the mastoid bone, and is more correctly termed a subperiosteal abscess of the mastoid. There is an erythematous painful fluctuant swelling behind the ear, which pushes the pinna forward (**Figure 9.2**). A CT scan is of benefit to exclude a co-existent intracranial collection. Treatment is with intravenous antibiotics, or mastoidectomy in cases that fail to settle.

Table 9.1. Complications of acute otitis media and their treatment. The more common complications are towards the top of the table.

Type	Notes	Treatment
Tympanic membrane perforation	Usually heals spontaneously	Topical antibiotics
Mastoiditis	Subperiosteal mastoid abscess	Antibiotics, mastoidectomy
Venous sinus thrombosis	Risk of propagation of thrombus	Antibiotics, ?anticoagulants, ?mastoidectomy
Temporal lobe abscess	Headache, fever, seizures or focal neurology	Antibiotics, drainage
Meningitis	Direct spread to meninges or through venous channels	Antibiotics, ?mastoidectomy
Facial palsy	May relate to dehiscence of facial nerve	Antibiotics
Gradenigo syndrome	Spread to the petrous apex of the temporal bone. Otorrhoea, abducent nerve palsy, facial pain	Antibiotics
Suppurative labyrinthitis	Vertigo and dead ear	Antibiotics, ?steroids,
Bezold's abscess	Spread of infection deep to sternomastoid muscle	Antibiotics, mastoidectomy
Luc's abscess	Spread of infection deep to temporalis muscle	Antibiotics, mastoidectomy
Otitis hydrocephalus	Cause uncertain	Supportive

OTITIS MEDIA WITH EFFUSION

OME describes the presence of a non-purulent effusion in the middle ear. It is more commonly called 'glue ear' because the effusion is often very tenacious, and in this respect resembles liquid glue.

Transient middle ear effusions are common during early childhood; OME is estimated to affect 75% of children in their second year of life. Many cases of OME occur following a preceding episode of AOM. However, some cases of OME occur *de novo*, for reasons that are incompletely understood, but may reflect subclinical infection of the middle ear.

If children who develop new-onset OME are followed, the majority of effusions will resolve within a few days or weeks (**Figure 9.3**). However, in a minority of cases, the effusion persists, and once present over 3 months is termed chronic OME (COME). If an effusion has been present for 3 months, then the chance of resolution is small in the short to medium term. Of all children presenting to an ENT clinic with effusion of unknown duration, fewer than half will resolve over the next 3 months.

COME affects 6–7% of 2-year old children. It can cause conductive hearing loss (although not necessarily so) and associated educational and linguistic difficulties in the short term. Opinion is divided as to the long-term consequences to an individual with COME, which in turn causes controversy over the necessity of treating COME in childhood.

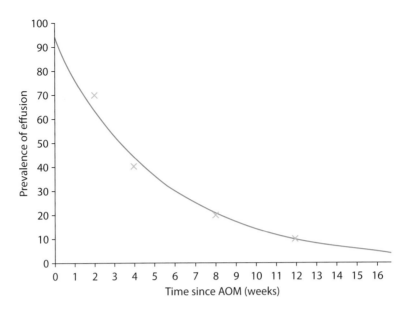

Figure 9.3. Presence of otitis media with effusion following an episode of acute otitis media. Resolution of effusion shows exponential decay. After 3 months (13 weeks) the disease is called chronic otitis media with effusion.

COME should be suspected in a child who fails to hear or who has educational or linguistic difficulties. It is more common in some conditions – Down syndrome, cleft palate, craniosynostosis or primary ciliary dyskinesia. In the non-syndromic child, risk factors are the same as those for AOM. Again, there is little evidence to support a difference in the anatomy or function of the ET in these children.

Otoscopy in OME reveals effusion deep to an intact TM (**Figure 9.4**), imparting a blue or a yellow hue to the middle ear. A type B tympanogram confirms the diagnosis, and an age-appropriate audiogram will characterise any associated hearing loss. In adults with unilateral glue ear, examination of the nasopharynx is necessary to exclude a carcinoma.

Recommendations in England are that treatment of COME should only be considered in cases that have lasted at least 3 months and where the auditory threshold is worse that 25 dB in both ears. In reality, the estimated disability from the hearing loss is the most important factor in deciding whether treatment is warranted.

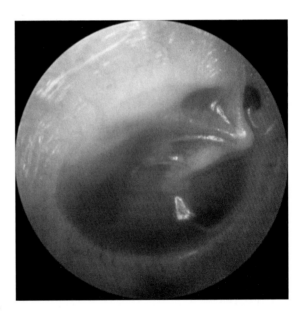

Figure 9.4. Otoscopic view of otitis media with effusion. Effusion is visible deep to an intact tympanic membrane. In this case there is also an air bubble and mild retraction of the tympanic membrane. (Courtesy David Pothier)

The most common treatment for COME is grommet insertion or a hearing aid. Grommets eliminate middle ear effusion while *in situ*, although how they do this is debated.

There is no evidence to support the use of antihistamines, antibiotics, nasal decongestants or nasal steroids to treat COME. There may be benefit from autoinflation of the ear, and commercially available devices for this purpose include the Otovent® Balloon and the EarPopper®.

Approximately 1 in 5 children treated with grommets have recurrence of their effusion once the grommet extrudes. A concurrent adenoidectomy may help to prevent further recurrence in those children having a second set of grommets.

FURTHER READING

Bhutta MF (2014) Epidemiology and pathogenesis of otitis media: construction of a phenotype landscape. *Audiol Neurootol* **19(3)**:210–223.

National Institute for Health and Clinical Excellence (2008) *Surgical Management of Otitis Media with Effusion in Children*. National Institute for Health and Clinical Excellence, Manchester.

www.thecochranelibrary.com (search for 'otitis media')

10
RETRACTION POCKETS AND PERFORATIONS

Peter Monksfield

Contents

INTRODUCTION

Abnormalities of the eardrum are common and often present at the time of, or subsequent to, an ear infection. A perforation in the eardrum presenting acutely after trauma or an infection will undergo spontaneous repair in up to 80% of cases.[1] White patches in the eardrum, called tympanosclerosis, which are due to collagen formation and also often contain calcium, are a sign of previous trauma or perforation and are not usually associated with hearing loss. However, tympanosclerosis can be present within the middle ear following repeated infections and cause a conductive hearing loss if it affects the function of the ossicular chain.

In those cases that do not undergo spontaneous repair and have a persisting abnormality, either with a retraction or a perforation, some may be asymptomatic with normal hearing. However, depending on the size and site of the abnormality in the eardrum, most will have some degree of conductive hearing loss. In those with long-standing perforations or retraction pockets and a history of repeated infections, there may also be some added underlying sensorineural hearing impairment, which is attributed to the repeated infections.

AETIOLOGY

Tympanic membrane (TM) perforations occur most commonly following trauma or an ear infection. They can also be iatrogenic such as following

ear syringing or subsequent to ventilation tube insertion.

A retraction pocket can form due to Eustachian tube dysfunction (ETD) or repeated bouts of inflammation.[2] Long-term negative pressure from ETD sucks the eardrum inwards. A retraction pocket may in advanced cases lead to the formation of a cholesteatoma. It is also thought that infection in a retraction pocket can then lead to a perforation of the TM.

CLASSIFICATION

Perforations can be classified by their size and by their location within the TM. The size of perforation can be described as a percentage of the size of the drum.[3] Perforations are central or marginal. Central perforations have a definite rim of membrane around the whole perforation (**Figure 10.1**) and occur within the eardrum. These are also called 'safe' perforations in that they are much less likely to be associated with an underlying cholesteatoma. Marginal perforations are 'unsafe' as they are in continuity with the bony margin of the tympanic ring and are more likely to occur in conjunction with a cholesteatoma in the middle ear and mastoid (**Figure 10.2**).

Retraction can occur in the pars tensa, the pars flaccida, or both. A grading system for pars tensa retraction pockets was described by Sadé[4] in 1979 (**Figure 10.3**):

Grade I: retracted TM.
Grade II: retraction with contact onto incus.
Grade III: retraction of TM onto the promontory, but mobile.
Grade IV: adhesive otitis media, TM retracted onto the promontory and fixed.

Clinically, grades III and IV can be distinguished by asking the patient to Valsalva and observing whether the eardrum moves away from the promontory.

Tos[5] described a grading system for retractions of the pars flaccida (**Figure 10.4**):

Grade I: pars flaccida not in contact with the malleus neck.
Grade II: pars flaccida in contact with the malleus neck.

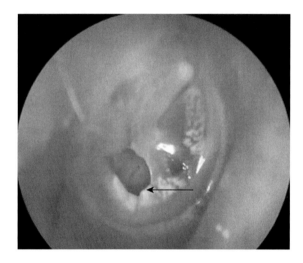

Figure 10.1. Central perforation with some minor tympanosclerosis in the eardrum (arrow).

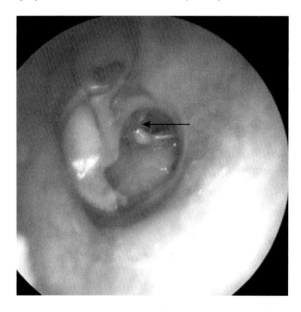

Figure 10.2. Marginal perforation with loss of the incus long process (arrow).

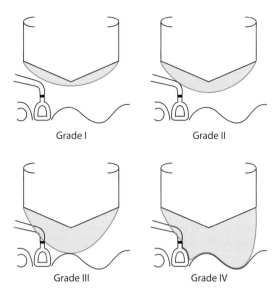

Grade I   Grade II

Grade III   Grade IV

Figure 10.3. Sadé pars tensa retraction grading.

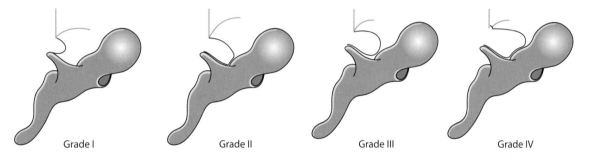

Grade I   Grade II   Grade III   Grade IV

Figure 10.4. Tos pars flaccida retraction grading.

Grade III: limited outer attic wall erosion.
Grade IV: severe outer attic wall erosion.

Retraction pockets once attached to the ossicular chain can cause some erosion of the chain. Commonly, pars tensa retractions of Sadé grade II and above cause erosion of the incus long process and loss of the incudostapedial joint (**Figure 10.5**), thereby reducing the function of the ossicular chain and causing a conductive hearing loss.

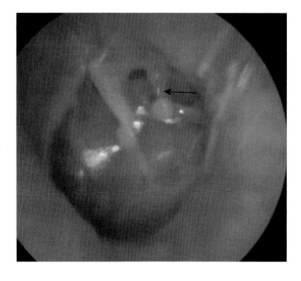

Figure 10.5. Posterior eardrum retraction with erosion of incus long process and only a fibrous attachment to the stapes (arrow).

SYMPTOMS

The symptoms associated with both retraction pockets and perforations are predominantly hearing loss and recurrent infections. They may also be asymptomatic. The hearing loss tends to be conductive in nature and can range from a mild impairment through to a maximal conductive hearing loss with an air–bone gap of up to 60 dB, seen in cases where there is ossicular damage and or fixation.

The size of the perforation, as well as the middle ear volume, plays a part in determination of the degree of hearing loss.[6] Larger perforations and smaller middle ear volumes tend to have a greater conductive hearing loss and larger air–bone gap. The hearing loss tends to be greater in the lower frequencies. Although it is thought that posterior perforations have greater hearing loss due to a phase cancellation effect on the round window membrane, only a small non-significant difference in hearing is seen between anterior and posterior perforations.[6]

Infection is usually characterised by ear discharge. This can be related to exposure of the ear to water during swimming or bathing. An increased rate of infection is seen in conditions of impaired immunity such as diabetes. Also, nutritional and environmental factors are implicated in recurrent ear infection.[3]

Other less common symptoms include tinnitus, disequilibrium and vertigo with a caloric effect from water or cold air exposure and rarely pain.

TREATMENT

Treatment for both retraction pockets and TM perforations is either conservative management or surgical intervention. Conservative management comprises avoiding water exposure to the ear and the use of hearing aids to treat hearing loss. This is appropriate in asymptomatic patients with normal hearing and stable retractions who are able to observe water precautions. The use of topical antibiotic therapy in infective episodes along with aural toilet is also advised. In those patients with a history of recurrent infections, progressive retractions or a significant conductive hearing loss, surgery should be considered.

Tympanoplasty is surgery for perforations and comprises the placement of some form of autologous or synthetic graft under or within the perforation. The most commonly used grafts are autologous materials such as temporalis fascia, cartilage or perichondrium. Surgery is usually performed under general anaesthesia and the graft is placed within the middle ear underneath the perforation (**Figure 10.6**). The ossicular chain is also assessed and surgical reconstruction can be

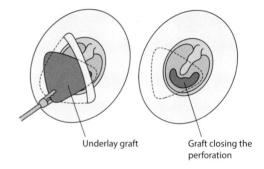

Underlay graft

Graft closing the perforation

Figure 10.6. Underlay tympanoplasty.

undertaken to improve the hearing (see Chapter 13: Ossiculoplasty). Many surgeons will define success of surgery as an intact TM. Rates of success quoted in the literature vary from 60–99%.[1] Typically, a success rate of over 80% would be considered acceptable for a surgeon performing this procedure.

The use of ventilation tubes may be tried in early retractions that have a mobile TM. Where this fails, or as an alternative, a tympanoplasty is required. The pocket needs to be elevated off the middle ear structures, as any squamous epithelium left within the middle ear will result in a cholesteatoma. The pocket is excised, thereby creating a perforation, with reconstruction of both the TM and ossicular chain performed in the same manner as with a perforation. Cartilage is advised to reconstruct the defect as a more rigid material reduces the chance of a recurrent retraction. High success rates are seen with this approach with over 80% showing no recurrent retraction at 12 months.[7]

SUMMARY

Chronic otitis media with perforation or retraction of the TM is a common problem and comprises a large part of the work of an ENT surgeon with an interest in otology. Many patients can be managed conservatively, particularly those with inactive retractions. However, a surgical approach should always be considered for patients that are symptomatic.

REFERENCES

1 Aggarwal R, Green KJM (2006) Myringoplasty. *J Laryngol Otol* **120**:429–432.
2 Nankivell PC, Pothier DD (2010) Surgery for tympanic membrane retraction pockets. *Cochrane Database Syst Rev* **Issue 7**. doi 10.1002/14651858.CD007943.pub2
3 Browning GG, Merchant SN, Kelley G *et al.* (2008) Chronic otitis media. In: *Scott-Brown's Otorhinolaryngology, Head and Neck Surgery*, 7th edn. (ed. M Gleeson) Hodder Arnold, London, pp. 3395–3445.
4 Sadé J (1979) The atelectatic ear. In: *Monograms in Clinical Otolaryngology, Secretory Otitis Media and its Sequelae.* (ed. J Sadé) Churchill Livingstone, New York, pp. 64–88.
5 Tos M, Poulsen G (1980) Attic retractions following secretory otitis. *Acta Oto-Laryngologica* **89**:479–486.
6 Ritvik P, Mehta RP, Rosowski JJ, Voss SE *et al.* (2006) Determinants of hearing loss in perforations of the tympanic membrane. *Otol Neurotol* **27**:136–143.
7 Spielmann P, Mills R (2006) Surgical management of retraction pockets of the pars tensa with cartilage and perichondrial grafts. *J Laryngol Otol* **120**:725–729.

11 CHOLESTEATOMA

Thomas P.C. Martin

Contents

DEFINITION AND CLASSIFICATION

A cholesteatoma is an expanding, destructive lesion of the temporal bone consisting of keratinising squamous epithelium. The condition is further classified aetiologically as either congenital or acquired and by anatomical location.

EPIDEMIOLOGY

Cholesteatoma is rare, with an incidence estimated at 1 per 10,000, an equal sex distribution and a peak incidence in the second decade of life.[1] Disease in children is recognised to be more extensive and aggressive, possibly due to immature Eustachian tube function. In common with other forms of chronic ear disease, it is more common in lower socioeconomic classes.[2]

PATHOGENESIS

▌ Congenital cholesteatoma

This is defined as a keratin cyst found behind a normal tympanic membrane (TM) and represents less than 1% of cholesteatomas. Congenital cholesteatomas are thought to arise either from the presence of an ectopic epidermis rest or from metaplasia. Their most common location is in the anterior mesotympanum where they are described as a Michael's body.

▌ Acquired cholesteatoma

Primary and secondary

The exact aetiology of primary cholesteatoma is debated but the most commonly accepted theory is that of progression of a retraction pocket of the TM, usually either in the pars flaccida (the 'attic' region superior to the lateral process of the malleus: 'primary cholesteatoma') or in the posterior segment of the pars tensa ('secondary cholesteatoma'). The alteration of normal anatomy interferes with squamous migration and leads to an aggregation of keratinous debris within the pocket. This leads to a chronic inflammatory process that stimulates squamous proliferation and expansion of the lesion with a peripheral osteoclastic activity eroding neighbouring temporal bone structures.[4] There is not a good understanding of why some retraction pockets progress to cholesteatoma while others do not.

Tertiary

A tertiary cholesteatoma is considered to be caused by iatrogenic or traumatic implantation of squamous epithelium into the middle ear (e.g. after grommet insertion or tympanoplasty). This classification is summarised in **Table 11.1**.

SYMPTOMS AND PRESENTATION

The most common symptoms are chronic otorrhoea and a conductive hearing loss (most commonly due to erosion of the lenticular process of the incus bone). Other symptoms may occur such as vertigo

Table 11.1. Meyerhoff and Truelson classification of cholesteatoma.[3]

Primary acquired	Arising from defect of the pars flaccida
Secondary acquired	Arising from a defect of the pars tensa
Tertiary acquired	Occurring behind an intact eardrum as a result of implantation or middle ear inflammation
Congenital	Probably arising from a nidus of trapped squamous epithelium present at birth

due to erosion of the lateral semicircular canal, facial nerve weakness due to destruction of bone covering the facial nerve or, rarely, a sensorineural hearing loss due to invasion of the cochlea. Occasionally, a cholesteatoma will present as an emergency with intracranial complications of sigmoid sinus thrombosis or extradural, subdural or intracerebral abscess. In these cases, management requires urgent treatment in collaboration with a neurosurgeon.

DIAGNOSIS

▊ Audiometry

A pure tone audiogram with both air and masked bone conduction is essential to assess hearing in both the affected and contralateral ear.

▊ Computed tomography

The diagnosis of cholesteatoma is made clinically but CT scanning can aid surgical planning. It should be recognised that keratin is indistinguishable from mucosal inflammation or effusion within the middle ear or mastoid: disease extent is gauged by evidence of bone erosion. CT can usefully demonstrate erosion of the otic capsule, the tegmen tympani, the fallopian canal and the bone covering the sigmoid sinus. Importantly, in a few rare cases, a CT scan may demonstrate a lesion extending medially to the petrous apex. These cases will often require treatment by a neurotologist.

▊ Magnetic resonance imaging

MRI may be often used postoperatively to assess rates of residual disease following intact canal wall surgery (see below).

MANAGEMENT/TREATMENT

▊ Examination

The microscope should be used to remove keratin and assess the extent of disease. It is important to recognise that a large cholesteatoma may arise from a very small attic defect, which can be covered by debris. Removal of such 'attic crusts' may be painful and require a general anaesthetic in children. The contralateral ear should always be examined.

▊ Surgery

The surgical principles to be followed are threefold:

- Definitive removal of squamous epithelium from the site of disease.
- Reconstruction of a stable neotympanum.
- Reconstruction of the hearing mechanism where possible.

The means by which this can be achieved fall into three basic categories: intact canal wall surgery ('combined approach tympanoplasty'), canal wall down ('modified radical mastoidectomy') or canal wall down surgery with reconstruction. The basic principles describing these operative approaches are illustrated below (**Figures 11.1A–F**). The different approaches and their perceived strengths and weaknesses are outlined in **Table 11.2**. A surgeon's approach will be guided by his or her experience and training and by patient factors. Few surgeons would dispute that outcomes are to a large extent dependent on individual surgical technique and that an effective outcome can be achieved using any one of the three methods described. These factors make objective comparisons between techniques difficult.

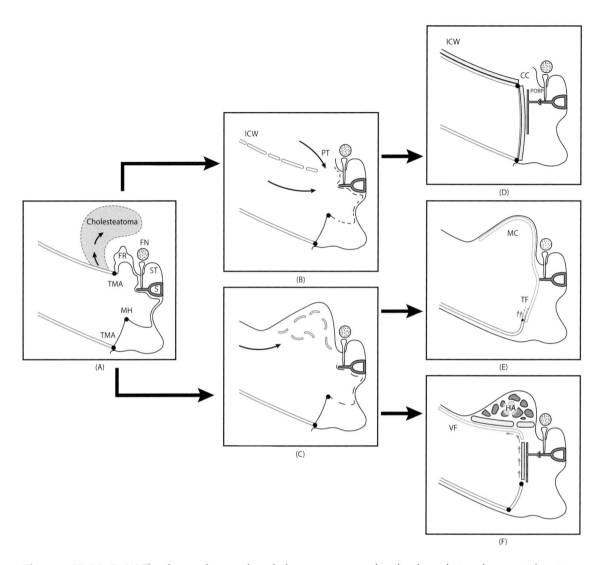

Figures 11.1A–F. (A) The diseased ear with a cholesteatoma extending backwards into the mastoid cavity. (B) A 'canal wall up' or 'combined approach' technique to remove the cholesteatoma through the middle ear and the mastoid via the posterior tympanotomy. (C) 'Canal wall down' or 'modified radical mastoidectomy'. The canal wall is drilled away to allow the surgeon to access disease in the mastoid. (D) Combined approach tympanoplasty. Creation of a neotympanum using cartilage. The malleus has been removed. (E) Modified radical mastoidectomy. Reconstruction with a mastoid cavity. Temporalis fascia covers exposed bone, leaving a smooth cavity, which becomes epithelialised. (F) Modified radical mastoidectomy with reconstruction of the canal wall/primary cavity obliteration. Cavity reconstruction using hydroxyapetite, cartilage and a vascularised flap, usually from the pericranium. **Key:** CC, conchal cartilage; FN, facial nerve; FR, facial recess; HA, hydroxyapetite; ICW, intact canal wall; MC, mastoid cavity; MH, malleus handle; PT, posterior tympanotomy; S, stapes; PORP, partial ossicular reconstruction prosthesis; ST, sinus tympani; TMA, tympanic membrane annulus; TF, temporalis fascia; VF, vascularised flap.

Table 11.2. Strengths and weaknesses of different surgical techniques.

	Recurrent disease[a]	Residual disease[b]	Hearing reconstruction	Infection
Combined approach tympanoplasty	Should be low risk if neotympanum stable, but this can be difficult in cases where negative middle ear pressures exist	May be present if disease located in places that are difficult to access. Reconstruction of neotympanum will usually hide residual disease	Should be good: posterior tympanotomy allows for good visualisation of prosthesis position and normal middle ear anatomy should allow for re-ventilation	Low risk if neotympanum stable
Modified radical mastoidectomy	Disease exteriorisation should lead to migration of keratin into cavity and out through external auditory canal	Risk of residual disease should be reduced by greater access to sinus tympani and facial recess during surgery	May be good but narrow middle ear cleft may reduce chances of good middle ear ventilation	Can be problematic if cavity irregular, external auditory meatus narrow or neotympanum perforated
Modified radical mastoidectomy with canal wall reconstruction	Recurrence should be minimised, as in modified radical mastoidectomy, but epithelial migration may be impaired if reconstruction not successful	Residual disease may be covered by reconstruction	May be good but narrow middle ear cleft may reduce chances of good middle ear ventilation	Should be low risk if reconstruction is effective

[a] Recurrent disease is defined as a cholesteatoma that forms from a new retraction pocket in the neotympanum.

[b] Residual disease is defined as cholesteatoma that forms from keratin not removed during the primary procedure.

ON-GOING MANAGEMENT

■ Combined approach tympanoplasty

Many surgeons advocate routine 'second look' surgery at 1 year to identify residual disease, which will be found in some 15% of operated ears, with rates higher in a paediatric population. This can often be achieved without disturbing the middle ear reconstruction; an endoscope can be used to view the middle ear through the posterior tympanotomy.

Alternatively, non-EPI diffusion-weighted MRI can be used to look for residual disease (see Chapter 5: Imaging of the ear); this technique can reliably identify cholesteatomas measuring >2–5 mm.[5] Diffusion-weighted MRI may also be used to exclude residual disease in primarily reconstructed modified radical cavities, although some surgeons argue that greater confidence in removing disease at primary surgery renders this investigation unnecessary.

▌▌ Modified radical mastoidectomy

Some modified radical mastoidectomy cavities will often require regular microsuction in order to remove keratin that collects in the cavity due to disrupted migration. The burden on patients created by ongoing aural toilet was one of the principle motivations for the development of intact canal wall tympanomastoidectomy.

▌▌ Mastoid revision

In some cases, mastoid cavities fail to heal effectively and lead to chronic infection, sometimes with recurrent cholesteatoma. The factors outlined in **Table 11.2** may contribute to this and further surgery should be guided by those problematic qualities. Mastoid revision may require meatoplasty, mastoid cavity obliteration, tympanoplasty or a combination of these procedures.

▌▌ Conservative

While most treatment is surgical, it is important to recognise that a small proportion of (usually elderly) patients with medical comorbidities that preclude surgery may instead need to be managed with regular aural toilet and topical treatment with combination antibiotic and steroid drops or ointments.

REFERENCES

1 Harker LA (1977) Cholesteatoma: an incidence study. In: *First International Conference on Cholesteatoma, Birmingham, Alabama.* (eds. BF McCabe, J Sadé, M Abramson) Aesculapius Publishing Company, pp. 308–309.
2 Khalid-Raja M, Tikka T, Coulson C (2014) Cholesteatoma: a disease of the poor (socially deprived)? *Eur Arch Otolaryngology* **272(10):**2799–2805.
3 Meyerhoff WL, Truelson J (1986) Cholesteatoma staging. *Laryngoscope* **96(9):**935–939.
4 Kuo CL (2014) Etiopathogenesis of acquired cholesteatoma: prominent theories and recent advances in biomolecular research. *Laryngoscope* **125(1):**234–240.
5 Jindal M, Riskella A, Jiang D *et al.* (2011) A systematic review of diffusion-weighted magnetic resonance imaging in the assessment of postoperative cholesteatoma. *Otol Neurotol* **32(8):**1243–1249.

12 OTOSCLEROSIS

Jeremy Lavy

Contents

INTRODUCTION

Otosclerosis is a condition affecting the bone of the otic capsule. In the disease process, the normal dense bone surrounding the labyrinth is replaced by a more cellular woven bone. Any part of the otic capsule can be involved but the commonest sites are just anterior to the oval window (the fissula ante fenestram) and in the region of the round window. Because the new diseased bone is less dense the condition is often referred to as otospongiosis by European specialists.

GENETICS

The true genetics would appear to be quite complex, although it can be partially explained as autosomal dominant with incomplete penetrance.

INCIDENCE

There is a quite a marked racial variation with European Caucasians being much more frequently affected than Afro-Caribbeans. Postmortem studies show an incidence of up to 10% in some populations, although it is likely that only one in ten of these would present clinically. The sex distribution is likely to be equal; however, the effect of hormonal changes during pregnancy on bone metabolism results in more rapid progression and so presents more frequently in women. Patients commonly present in their 30's and 40's.

SYMPTOMS

At first presentation the commonest finding is of a conductive hearing loss. This can be unilateral or bilateral. Tinnitus is also often present. The presence of vertigo may indicate a secondary endolymphatic hydrops, which is commonly felt to be a contraindication to surgery. The natural history is for the degree of hearing loss to progress. This is initially due to a progression of the conductive component but more latterly can also reflect an increasing sensorineural element.

DIFFERENTIAL DIAGNOSIS

In patients with an intact drum and a conductive loss the following should also be considered:

- Congenital ossicular fixation: consider if hearing loss dates back to childhood.
- Adhesive otitis media: enquire about history of recurrent ear infections.
- Ossicular discontinuity: usually associated with trauma.
- Osteogenesis imperfecta: enquire about other fractures, look for blue sclera.
- Tympanosclerosis: carefully inspect eardrum for sclerotic patches.
- Superior semicircular canal dehiscence: may be noted on CT scanning.

DIAGNOSIS

The otoscopic appearance of the eardrum is classically completely normal. Tuning fork tests will show a conductive hearing loss (bone conduction louder than air and a midline tuning fork lateralising to the worse affected ear).

A pure tone audiogram is essential (**Figure 12.1**). The masked bone conduction thresholds may be falsely elevated (the so-called Carrhart effect), particularly at 2 kHz. A tympanogram is also advisable to avoid missing one of the commonest causes of a conductive loss – a middle ear effusion (glue ear). The diagnosis can be confirmed by a CT scan of the temporal bone, although this is not essential (**Figure 12.2**). Studies show around a 90% sensitivity and specificity for CT as a diagnostic tool for otosclerosis.[1]

MANAGEMENT

There are two different treatment options:

- Some form of hearing aid: conventional hearing aid, bone conductor aid, surgically implantable aid (bone-anchored hearing aid or other surgical bone conductor).
- Surgery to re-establish the chain of vibration from the drum to the cochlear: stapedectomy

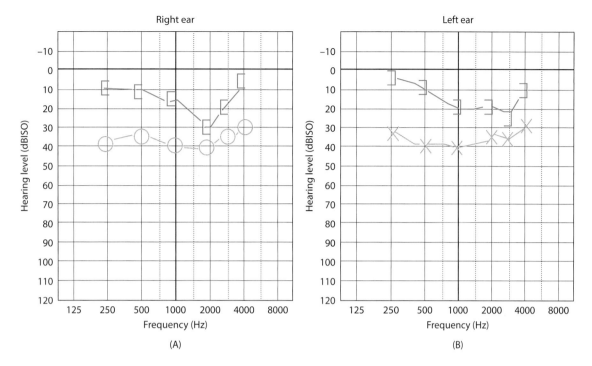

Figure 12.1. A classic 'otosclerosis' audiogram.

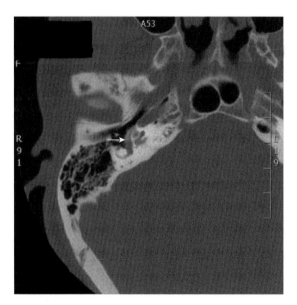

Figure 12.2. CT scan showing lucency (otospongiosis) around the cochlea and extending onto the stapes footplate (arrow).

(where the whole stapes footplate is removed), stapedotomy (where the footplate is left *in situ* and a fenestration is made through it) and the historical fenestration operation where the bone over the lateral semicircular canal is removed to expose a small area of membranous labyrinth.

The commonest surgical intervention is now stapedotomy.[2] Surgery can be performed down the ear canal and is eminently suitable for local anaesthesia. A flap, comprising posterior canal wall skin and the eardrum, is elevated and folded forward. Once the diagnosis is confirmed the attachments of the stapes are divided (incudostapedial joint and stapedius tendon). With the help of a laser, the posterior crus of the stapes is divided and the anterior crus can then be down fractured and the stapes superstructure removed. A small (0.4–0.8 mm) stapedotomy is fashioned through the mid portion of the footplate (**Figure 12.3**) and a piston of appropriate length is inserted into the fenestration and then attached to the long process of the incus (**Figure 12.4**).

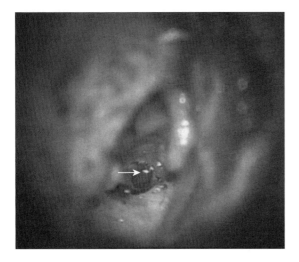

Figure 12.3. Operative view of a stapedotomy in the right ear (arrow).

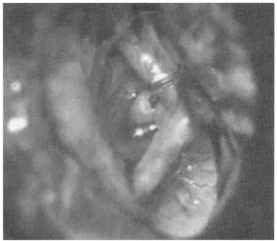

Figure 12.4. Operative view of a stapes piston *in situ*.

Closure of the air–bone gap is achievable in >90% of patients with an experienced surgeon. Complications include transient dizziness, altered taste on the side of the tongue (relating to manipulation of the chorda tympani) and dead ear (complete loss of hearing and balance function). The incidence of this catastrophic complication should be <1%. Revision surgery is indicated where there is recurrence of the conductive loss. This can be due to dislocation of the prosthesis, too tight a stapedotomy or occasionally fibrosis developing around the prosthesis.

In advanced end stage otosclerosis, where there is insufficient cochlear reserve to consider stapes surgery, cochlear implantation can be considered. There are two issues in this regard: firstly, there is a risk of cochlear duct obliteration by the disease process and so an MRI scan should always be obtained; and secondly, the loss of mineralised bone around the cochlear can result in spread of current and symptoms of non-auditory stimulation such as pain and facial twitching.

REFERENCES

1 Virk JS1, Singh A, Lingam RK (2013) The role of imaging in the diagnosis and management of otosclerosis. *Otol Neurotol* **34(7):**e55–60.
2 Vincent R, Sperling NM, Oates J *et al.* (2006) Surgical findings and long-term hearing results in 3,050 stapedotomies for primary otosclerosis: a prospective study with the otology-neurotology database. *Otol Neurotol* **27(8 Suppl 2):**S25–47.

13 OSSICULOPLASTY

Simon Lloyd

Contents

INTRODUCTION

The ossicular chain consists of three ossicles: the malleus, incus and stapes. These articulate with each other via diarthrodial joints. The function of the ossicular chain is to optimise the transfer of acoustic energy from the environment, via the tympanic membrane to the cochlea.[1]

Dysfunction of the chain results in a conductive hearing loss and this may result from fixation, erosion or subluxation of the ossicles. The common causes of primary ossicular dysfunction are summarised in **Table 13.1**.

This chapter describes the common diseases that affect the ossicular chain, methods by which

ossicular dysfunction occurs and the techniques by which ossicular function can be restored. Otosclerosis is not discussed, as this is the subject of a separate chapter.

Table 13.1. Common causes of ossicular dysfunction.

- Otosclerosis
- Ossicular erosion
- Tympanosclersosis
- Fibrous adhesions
- Traumatic subluxation
- Congenital fixation and malformation
- Joint ankylosis (e.g. rheumatoid arthritis)

AETIOLOGY

Chronic otitis media and recurrent acute otitis media are the commonest causes of ossicular disease. These may result in fixation, through fibrosis or tympanosclerotic deposition, or erosion of the ossicular chain.

Acquired ankylosis of the ossicular joints may occur (e.g. as a result of systemic rheumatological disease). Similarly, congenital fixation or malformation of the ossicular chain may also rarely occur.

Erosion of the ossicular chain most often occurs at the long process of the incus or the stapes superstructure, as these have a poorer blood supply than other areas of the ossicular chain.[2]

Significant head injury or direct trauma to the middle ear can result in subluxation of one or more of the ossicles, the incus being the most commonly affected. It is also possible for fracture of one or more of the ossicles to occur.

DIAGNOSIS

The diagnosis of ossicular chain dysfunction is based on the clinical history, the appearance of the tympanic membrane and the pure tone audiogram. Important points to identify are a history of previous middle ear disease, a history of previous head injury, middle ear trauma or surgery. Ossicular chain dysfunction is more common in the presence of a tympanic membrane perforation or retraction and tympanic membrane tympanosclerosis. Ossicular discontinuity or erosion may at times be clearly seen through a perforation in the tympanic membrane. In some cases, CT imaging of the ear may also be helpful, although this is not universally advocated.

TREATMENT

The need for treatment is determined by the severity of the hearing loss, the attitude of the patient to the different available interventions, the likely aetiology of the ossicular dysfunction, the status of the opposite ear and the preferences of the treating surgeon. Options include conservative management, traditional hearing aids, passive or active implantable bone anchored hearing aids, active middle ear implants or ossicular surgery. The following discussion will focus on ossicular surgery.

Numerous methods and materials for the surgical restoration of the structure and function of the ossicular chain have been described.[3] Autologous materials such as the incus, cortical bone or cartilage may be used. Alternatively, there are many types of prostheses, manufactured from alloplastic materials, that are available. Materials in common use include titanium[4] and hydroxyapetite. There are also hydroxyapatite and ionomeric cements available that can be used to reconstruct erosion of the long process of the incus. The advantages and disadvantages of autologous verses alloplastic materials are presented in **Table 13.2**.

▐ Ossicular chain erosion

When there is erosion of the ossicular chain, the most useful way of deciding on the type of reconstruction to perform is to consider where the defect lies.

Erosion of the long process of the incus

This type of defect may be reconstructed using an incudostapedial joint replacement prosthesis. These have a shoe or clip that fits over the remnant of the

Table 13.2. Advantages and disadvantges of autologous versus alloplastic ossicular reconstruction.

	Autologous	Alloplastic
Biocompatible	++	+
Readily available	+/−	++
Reliable outcomes	+	+
Ease of use	+	+
Risk of recurrent cholesteatoma	+/−	−

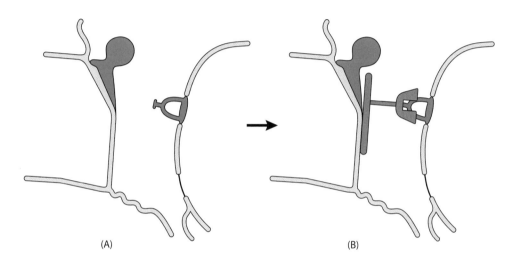

(A)   (B)

Figures 13.1A, B. Partial ossicular replacement prosthesis (PORP) for the reconstruction of the ossicular chain in the presence of an intact stapes superstructure. (A) The incus is absent but the stapes superstructure is intact. (B) The PORP is in place to replace the absent incus.

long process of the incus and a cup that sits on the head of the stapes. Alternatively, cement may be used to bridge the gap between incus and stapes superstructure.[5] Finally, the incus may be removed completely and a partial ossicular replacement prosthesis used (see below).

Stapes present

Alloplastic partial ossicular replacement prostheses (PORPs) have become the mainstay of ossicular reconstruction if the stapes is intact. The prosthesis consists of a head that is positioned under the tympanic membrane and a cup that is placed onto the stapes head with a shaft joining the two. A cartilage interposition graft between the head of

the prosthesis and the tympanic membrane may be required to minimize the risk of extrusion. The typical arrangement of a PORP within the middle ear is shown (**Figures 13.1A, B**).

Incus transposition is used by some surgeons. The incus is harvested and reshaped. It is then reinserted in a different configuration in order to restore ossicular continuity. The typical alterations made to the shape of the incus and the position in which the incus is placed once modified are shown (**Figures 13.2A–C**).

Autologous cartilage harvested from the pinna may also be used to reconstruct this type of defect, particularly if the middle ear is very shallow. A small square

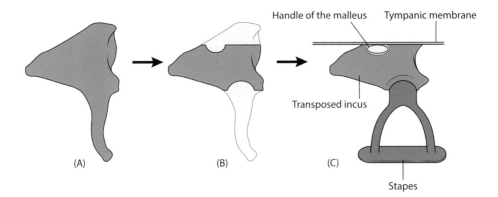

Handle of the malleus   Tympanic membrane

Transposed incus

Stapes

(A)   (B)   (C)

Figures 13.2A–C. Incus transposition. (A) The intact incus. (B) The modified incus. (C) The transposed incus in position.

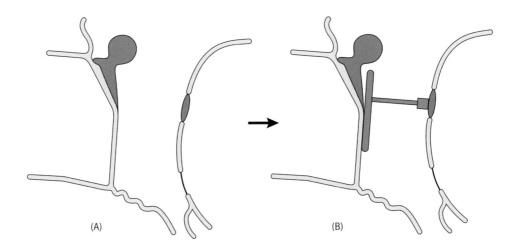

(A)   (B)

Figures 13.3A, B. Total ossicular replacement prosthesis (TORP) for the reconstruction of the ossicular chain in the absence of an intact stapes superstructure. (A) The incus and stapes superstructure are absent. (B) The TORP is in place to replace the absent incus and stapes superstructure.

of cartilage is placed between the stapes head and the tympanic membrane to produce a columellar effect.

Stapes absent

If the stapes is absent, the primary means of reconstruction is a total ossicular replacement prosthesis (TORP). The design is similar to that of a PORP but rather than a cup at the distal end there is a shoe that sits on the footplate of the stapes. As with the PORP, a cartilage interposition graft is also usually required. The typical arrangement of a TORP is shown (**Figures 13.3A, B**).

▮ Ossicular fixation

If fixation is the result of fibrous adhesions, it may be possible to divide these and restore the mobility of the ossicular chain. This may be performed using middle ear instruments or with the assistance of a laser.

If fixation is due to tympanosclerotic deposits, it is sometimes possible to separate these from the ossicular chain and restore its mobility. However, this can be difficult to achieve without significantly risking inner ear function.

Ankylosis of the malleoincudal joint or incudostapedial joint is best treated by dividing the incudostapedial joint and removing the incus. The ossicular chain can then be reconstructed using one of the techniques outlined above.

▌ Ossicular subluxation

It is not usually possible to restore the subluxed ossicle into its original position and it is therefore necessary to use one of the techniques outlined above to reconstruct the ossicular chain. The technique selected depends on the circumstances but a PORP or TORP are most frequently used.

OUTCOMES OF OSSICULOPLASTY

The outcome of ossicular surgery is dependent on a number of factors including the presence or absence of the stapes superstructure, the amount of inflammation or fibrosis in the middle ear, the depth of the middle ear cleft, the pneumatisation of the middle ear and the surgical technique employed.

Reconstruction in the presence of a stapes superstructure is generally more reliable than reconstruction when the superstructure is absent. Successful closure of the air–bone gap to within 15 dB of the opposite ear is the benchmark for success.[6] This is achievable in up to 70% of cases if the superstructure is present and in approximately 50% of cases if it is absent.[7]

CONCLUSION

There are a wide range of techniques available for the reconstruction of the ossicular chain, with partial or total ossicular replacement currently the most popular. The technique and type of reconstruction used needs to be tailored to the clinical circumstances. Despite the variety of options, outcomes are variable.

REFERENCES

1 Kurokawa H, Goode RL (1995) Sound pressure gain produced by the human middle ear. *Otolaryngol Head Neck Surg* **113:**349–355.
2 Chen H, Okumura T, Emura S *et al.* (2008) Scanning electron microscopic study of the human auditory ossicles. *Ann Anat* **190(1):**53–58.
3 Yung MW (2003) Literature review of alloplastic materials in ossiculoplasty. *J Laryngol Otol* **117(6):**431–436.
4 Zeitler DM, Lalwani AK (2010) Are postoperative hearing results better with titanium ossicular reconstruction prostheses? *Laryngoscope* **120(1):**2–3.
5 Watson GJ, Narayan S (2014) Bone cement: how effective is it at restoring hearing in isolated incudostapedial erosion? *J Laryngol Otol* **128(8):**690–693.
6 Browning GG, Gatehouse S, Swan IR (1991) The Glasgow Benefit Plot: a new method for reporting benefits from middle ear surgery. *Laryngoscope* **101(2):**180–185.
7 Truy E, Naiman AN, Pavillon C *et al.* (2007) Hydroxyapatite versus titanium ossiculoplasty. *Otol Neurotol* **28:**492–498.

14 BONE-ANCHORED HEARING AIDS

Philip J. Clamp

Contents

INTRODUCTION

Bone-anchored hearing aids (BAHAs) exploit the principle of bone conduction hearing, in which sound energy can be transmitted directly to the inner ear via the bones of the skull. Bone conduction hearing bypasses the outer and middle ear, circumventing anatomical or pathological problems in these areas.

BAHAs use titanium implants, surgically inserted into the skull. The bone around the implant forms a closely-knit interface, a process known as osseointegration. The bone-anchored fixture is then coupled to an external sound processor either directly through a percutaneous abutment or indirectly using transcutaneous magnets (**Figures 14.1A–C**).

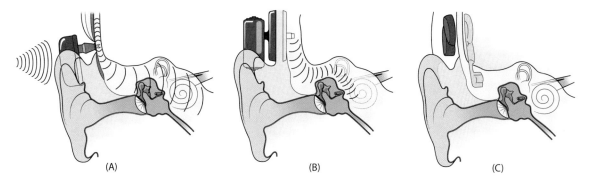

Figures 14.1A–C. Bone-anchored hearing aid (BAHA) types. (A) Directly coupled BAHA. (B) Magnetically coupled BAHA. (C) Active BAHA. Implanted component includes floating mass transducer.

BAHAs are useful for patients with a range of audiological and pathological conditions, in whom air-conduction hearing aids are not ideal.

Pathological indications include:

- Any patient requiring hearing aids in which air-conduction aids cannot be fitted (e.g. external ear canal atresia, microtia).
- Any patient in which air-conduction hearing aids exacerbate underlying conditions (e.g. otitis externa, open mastoid cavity infection, tympanic membrane perforation).

Audiological indications include:

- Conductive hearing loss with normal or near normal cochlear function (e.g. ear canal atresia, otosclerosis, tympanosclerosis, ossicular chain discontinuity, congenital conductive loss).
- Mixed hearing loss with mild to moderate underling sensorineural loss of less that 45–60 dbHL, depending on implant and processor type (e.g. chronic suppurative otitis media [CSOM], otosclerosis with cochlea involvement).

- Single-sided severe to profound sensorineural hearing loss (**Figure 14.2**); the BAHA is used to conduct sound to the contralateral ear (e.g. sudden idiopathic sensorineural hearing loss, vestibular schwannoma, temporal bone fracture, Ménière's disease).
- Patient preference for BAHA sound quality (typically for conductive losses greater than 35 dBHL).[1]

The commonest indication for BAHA is active chronic suppurative otitis media (COSM), in which patients with conductive or mixed hearing loss are unable to wear air-conduction hearing aids due to exacerbation of infections.[2] During patient evaluation for a BAHA, trial of a bone-conduction hearing aid on a headband is extremely useful in giving patients a realistic expectation of the sound quality that BAHAs can provide. Patients can be reassured, with a degree of certainly, that the sound quality of a BAHA will be the same or better than that provided by a non-invasive bone conduction aid. Each type of BAHA has different advantages and disadvantages (**Table 14.1**).

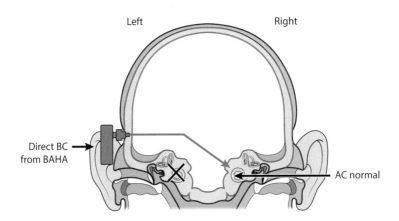

Figure 14.2. Bone-anchored hearing aid (BAHA) use in single-sided sensorineural hearing loss. BAHAs are used to to transmit sound from the deafened side to the contralateral ear, thus reducing the 'head-shadow' effect BC, bone conduction; AC, air conduction.

Table 14.1. Comparison of current bone-anchored hearing aid makes and models.

Implant type	Examples	Advantages	Disadvantages
Directly coupled	Baha Connect[a] Oticon Ponto[b]	Simple insertion technique. Suitable up to 45–60 dBHL BC depending on SP model	Requires ongoing abutment site care. Risk of soft tissue reactions and need for revision surgery. Higher likelihood of traumatic and infective implant loss. Percutaneous abutment may be cosmetically unacceptable to some
Magnetically coupled	Baha Attract[a] Sophono Alpha[c]	Minimal soft tissue reactions. No cosmetic issues when SP removed	Reduced power – only suitable for normal or mild loss in BC
Active implants	MED-EL Bonebridge[d]	Minimal soft tissue reactions. No cosmetic issues when SP removed. Suitable up to 45 dBHL BC	Large implant package requires surgical planning and deeper bone-well

[a] Cochlear Bone Anchored Solutions AB (Mölnlycke, Sweden); [b] Oticon Medical AB (Askim, Sweden); [c] Sophono (Boulder, USA); [d] MED-EL (Innsbruck, Austria); BC, bone conduction; SP, sound processor.

SURGICAL TECHNIQUE

BAHA implantation can be undertaken under general or local anaesthesia. For paediatric patients, bone maturity and skull thickness (minimum 3 mm required) limit the age of implantation to 3 years and over (not licensed under 5 years old in USA and Canada). A one-stage procedure, in which the bone-anchored fixture and percutaneous abutment are both implanted, is standard for adult patients (**Figures 14.3A–H**). A one- or two-stage procedure can be undertaken in children. A second bone-anchored fixture, without the percutaneous abutment ('sleeper' fixture), is often implanted simultaneously and acts as a backup if required.

The traditional approach of soft tissue reduction and skin splitting/grafting has, more recently, been replaced with a non-soft tissue reduction technique using longer abutments.[3] This technique appears to reduce the risk of soft tissue infections, as well as providing a more cosmetically acceptable implant site by preserving surrounding hair and scalp profile.

The site of implantation is usually postero-superior to the ear canal, in a position where the external sound processor will not contact the pinna. Consideration must be given to previous surgery, such as mastoidectomy for CSOM or craniotomy sites for vestibular schwannoma removal. In cases of aural atresia, skin that may be required for future cosmetic reconstruction of the pinna should not be violated.

Magnetically coupled or active devices are implanted as per the manufacturers' guidance, with elevation of a local scalp flap to avoid scars over the implant site.

In adults, sufficient osseointegration and wound healing have usually taken place by 4 weeks in order to allow loading of the external sound processor. In children, up to 3 months of osseointegration may be allowed before loading.

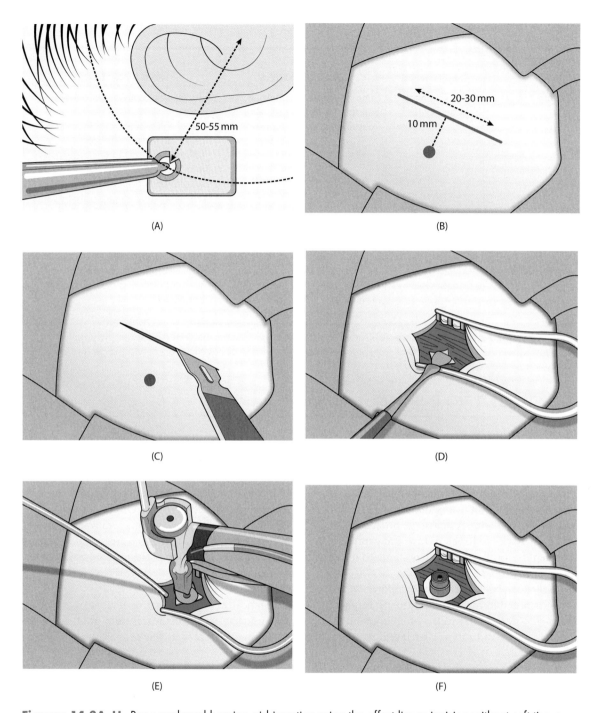

(A)

(B)

(C)

(D)

(E)

(F)

Figures 14.3A–H. Bone-anchored hearing aid insertion using the offset linear incision without soft tissue reduction. *(Continued)*

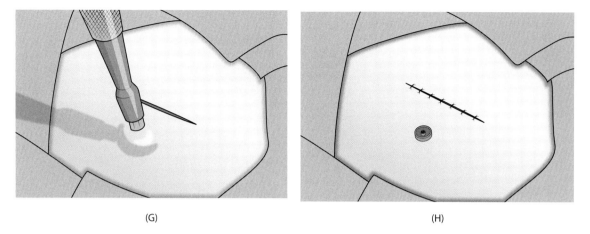

(G) (H)

Figures 14.3A–H. (Continued) Bone-anchored hearing aid insertion using the offset linear incision without soft tissue reduction.

COMPLICATIONS OF BONE-ANCHORED HEARING AIDS

The commonest complication of directly coupled BAHAs is local soft tissue reaction around the percutaneous abutment.[4] Up to 25% of patients experience some form of soft tissue problems, including skin irritation, granulations, tissue thickening/overgrowth and infection. Reactions are often temporary. Treatment requires careful wound care, cleaning and topical or systemic antibiotics. Around 10% of adult patients will require revision surgery to correct more persistent issues or replace failed implants. Complications are more common in children, with a higher rate of implant loss and extrusion mainly due in trauma or infection.[2] Magnetically coupled and active BAHAs do not have any skin penetrating components and thus complications are less. Local skin pressure may lead to discomfort requiring reduction in magnet strength or temporary cessation in use.[5]

REFERENCES

1 De Wolf MJ, Hendrix S, Cremers CW *et al.* (2011) Better performance with bone-anchored hearing aid than acoustic devices in patients with severe air-bone gap. *Laryngoscope* **121(3):**613–616.

2 Dun CA, Faber HT, de Wolf MJ *et al.* (2012) Assessment of more than 1,000 implanted percutaneous bone conduction devices: skin reactions and implant survival. *Otol Neurotol* **33(2):**192–198.

3 Husseman J, Szudek J, Monksfield P *et al.* (2013) Simplified bone-anchored hearing aid insertion using a linear incision without soft tissue reduction. *J Laryngol Otol* **127(Suppl 2):**S33–38.

4 Hobson JC, Roper AJ, Andrew R *et al.* (2010) Complications of bone-anchored hearing aid implantation. *J Laryngol Otol* **124(2):**132–136.

5 Sylvester DC, Gardner R, Reilly PG *et al.* (2013) Audiologic and surgical outcomes of a novel, nonpercutaneous, bone conducting hearing implant. *Otol Neurotol* **34(5):**922–926.

15

MIDDLE EAR IMPLANTS

Neil Donnelly

Contents

INTRODUCTION

The term middle ear implant describes a device placed within the middle ear in order to improve hearing. Middle ear implants (MEIs) are divided into active and passive. Passive devices are ossiculoplasty prostheses; their role is to attempt to restore middle ear mechanics. Active MEIs are surgically implanted 'hearing aids' that are directly coupled to either the ossicles or inner ear. Sound is converted to electrical energy and then transduced to mechanical energy to vibrate the ossicles or directly drive the cochlea via the round or oval windows.

INDICATIONS

▌ Sensorineural hearing loss

MEIs can rehabilitate sensorineural hearing losses ranging from mild to severe.[1,2] Suitable candidates include those with a hearing loss unable to wear conventional hearing aids due to recurrent infections or allergy. Suitable candidates need to fulfill the following criteria:

- Air–bone gap of ≤10 dB.
- Stable hearing loss.

- Speech understanding score of ≥50%.
- Normal middle ear anatomy and function.

The direct drive of the MEI has the following advantages over the indirect drive of conventional hearing aids:

- Elimination of occlusion effect.
- Reduced feedback.
- Improved high frequency sound fidelity.
- More natural sound quality.

▊ Conductive and mixed hearing loss

MEIs are able to rehabilitate a wide range of conductive or mixed hearing losses. Suitable mixed hearing or pure conductive losses may arise as a result of external auditory canal stenosis, external ear malformation[3], otosclerosis, middle ear disease[4] or lateral petrosectomy with blind sac closure.[5] Suitable candidates need to fulfill the following criteria:

- Stable bone conduction thresholds.
- A healthy middle ear space or closed middle ear with no active infection.

The advantages of the direct drive of a MEI over a bone conduction device in the presence of a mixed or conductive loss include:

- Improved speech in noise.
- Improved sound localisation.
- More natural sound quality.

ACTIVE MIDDLE EAR IMPLANTS

▊ MED-EL™ VIBRANT SOUNDBRIDGE®

The VIBRANT SOUNDBRIDGE® device (MED-EL UK) is used to rehabilitate sensorineural, conductive and mixed hearing losses. It consists of an external speech processor and an implanted receiver stimulator connecting to a vibrating ossicular prosthesis also known as the floating mass transducer (FMT) (**Figure 15.1**). The FMT is an electromagnetic transducer that attaches to the incus (short or long process), stapes or round

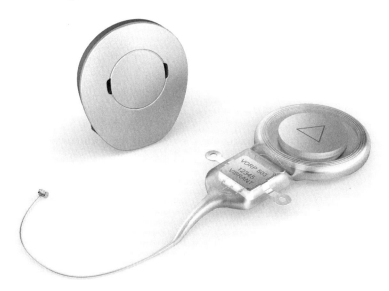

Figure 15.1. VIBRANT SOUNDBRIDGE® middle ear implant and SAMBA audio processor (courtesy of MED-EL UK Ltd).

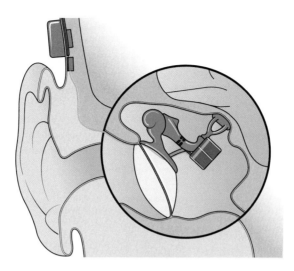

Figure 15.2. Middle ear implant attached to the long process of the incus.

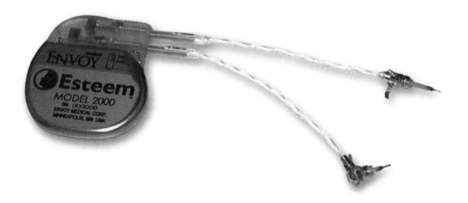

Figure 15.3. The fully implantable Esteem® Hearing Implant™ (courtesy of Envoy Medical Corporation, USA).

window via a range of customised couplers. The movement of the FMT augments the natural movement of the ossicles (by attachment to the incus (**Figure 15.2**) or stapes) or directly stimulates the inner ear via the round or oval windows.

▌ Envoy Esteem®

The Esteem® Hearing Implant™ (Envoy Medical Corporation, USA) is used to rehabilitate sensorineural hearing losses. It is a totally implantable device with a battery life of 5–9 years. The implant has two leads that extend into the middle

ear (**Figure 15.3**). The procedure requires a portion of the incus to be removed. The sensor makes use of normal physiology and is cemented to the remaining portion of the incus to detect tympanic membrane motion. The device amplifies the signal and transmits this to the head of the stapes via the driver.

▌ Cochlear™ MET® and Carina® Systems

The MET® Middle Ear Implant System (Cochlear Boulder, USA) is indicated for moderate to severe sensorineural hearing loss and for moderate to severe mixed or conductive hearing loss. The Carina® Fully Implantable Middle Ear Implant System (Cochlear Boulder, USA) implant has the same indications as the MET® implant system but is fully implantable (**Figure 15.4**). In cases of sensorineural hearing loss, the actuator probe tip is coupled to the incus. In cases of mixed or conductive hearing loss, the actuator can be coupled to the stapes, oval window or round window by means of an actuator extension.

▮ Cochlear™ Codacs™ System

The Codacs™ Direct Acoustic Cochlear Implant System (Cochlear Limited, Australia) (**Figure 15.5**) is a more powerful implant system that rehabilitates severe to profound mixed hearing loss via direct mechanical stimulation of the cochlear fluid. The principal indication is otosclerosis, with the device being coupled with a standard stapedectomy prosthesis.

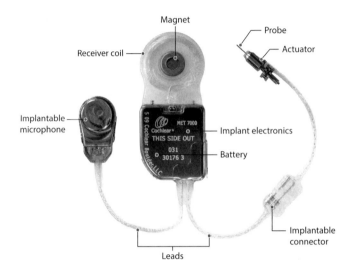

Figure 15.4. The Carina® implant system (courtesy of Cochlear Limited).

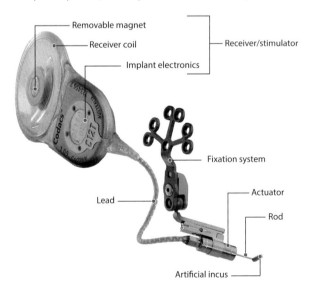

Figure 15.5. The Codacs™ implant system (courtesy of Cochlear Limited).

ASSESSMENT

Assessment is by a multidisciplinary team to determine candidacy and the potential benefits of a MEI.

OPERATION

A post-auricular approach is used. The incision is placed further posteriorly in cases of aural atresia to facilitate future reconstructive surgery of the pinna.[3] A cortical mastoidectomy is performed and the dissection continued forward into the root of the zygomatic process to provide good access for coupling to the head of the malleus and the body of the incus. It is imperative not to contact the ossicles with the drill while exposing this area to avoid the risk of further hearing loss.[6] An extended posterior tympanotomy is necessary for coupling to the long process of the incus, stapes, oval window or round window. The receiver stimulator is secured in a bony well or tight sub-periosteal pocket.

The majority of MEIs can be performed as day surgery procedures. Device activation is typically after 4–6 weeks.

MEIs are an excellent means of hearing rehabilitation in those individuals who do not receive adequate benefit from conventional hearing aids. Their application and indications continue to broaden. Long-term efficacy remains under investigation but studies suggest good functional and audiological outcomes[1,7] in addition to good cost effectiveness.[8]

REFERENCES

1 Butler CL, Thavaneswaran P, Lee IH (2013) Efficacy of the active middle-ear implant in patients with sensorineural hearing loss. *J Laryngol Otol* **127(Suppl):**S8–16.

2 Wagner F, Todt I, Wagner J *et al.* (2010) Indications and candidacy for active middle ear implants. *Adv Otorhinolaryngo.* **69:**20–26.

3 Agterberg MJH, Frenzel H, Wollenberg B *et al.* (2014) Amplification options in unilateral aural atresia: an active middle ear implant or a bone conduction device? *Otol Neurotol* **35(1):**129–135.

4 Luers JC, Huttenbrink K-B, Zahnert T *et al.* (2013) Vibroplasty for mixed and conductive hearing loss. *Otol Neurotol* **34(6):**1005–1012.

5 Henseler MA, Polanski JF, Schlegel C *et al.* (2014) Active middle ear implants in patients undergoing subtotal petrosectomy: long-term follow-up. *Otol Neurotol* **35(3):**437–441.

6 Jiang D, Bibas A, Santuli C *et al.* (2007) Equivalent noise level generated by drilling onto the ossicular chain as measured by laser Doppler vibrometry: a temporal bone study. *Laryngoscope* **117(6):**1040–1045.

7 Tysome JR, Moorthy R, Lee A *et al.* (2010) Systematic review of middle ear implants: do they improve hearing as much as conventional hearing AIDS? *Otol Neurotol* **31(9):**1369–1375.

8 Edfeldt L, Stromback K, Grendin J *et al.* (2014) Evaluation of cost-utility in middle ear implantation in the "Nordic School": a multicenter study in Sweden and Norway. *Acta Otolaryngol* **134(1):**19–25.

16 PRESBYACUSIS

Ruth V. Lloyd

Contents

DEFINITION

Presbyacusis, or age-related hearing loss, is an almost universal feature of ageing. Presbyacusis is derived from two Greek words: 'presbys' meaning elder and 'akousis' meaning hearing. It is not a disease, but rather a description of the changes affecting the auditory system as a person ages, resulting in a bilateral, sensorineural deafness.

PREVALENCE

The prevalence is of presbyacusis is high, with up to 70–80% of people older than 75 years affected.[1] Hearing aids are still underutilised and in a recent survey, only 22% of Americans over 80 with a known hearing loss wear hearing aids.[2]

CLINICAL FEATURES

The sensory hair cells in the cochlea that code for sounds higher than 3 kHz are the most vulnerable to damage, and therefore thresholds for these high frequencies start to increase first, followed by those of the middle and lower frequencies (**Figures 16.1A, B**). These changes occur gradually, often starting in middle age, and are usually symmetrical. The hearing loss is often noticed more by

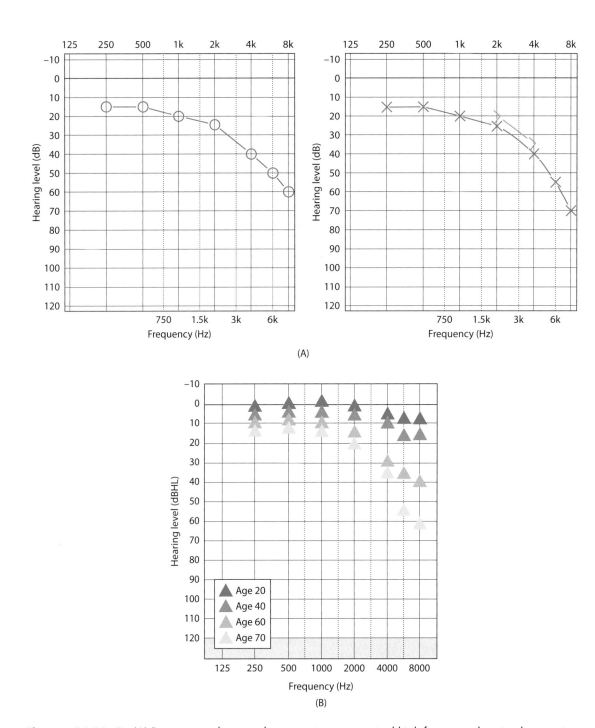

Figures 16.1A, B. (A) Pure tone audiogram demonstrating symmetrical high frequency hearing loss, typical of presbyacusis (male patient, aged 78). (B) Typical hearing thresholds for 'otologically normal' men at differing ages. Note that women's hearing tends to be slightly better across the frequencies, and that hearing thresholds for otologically unscreened populations (i.e. 'normal' hearing thresholds) are approximately 5 dB worse across the thresholds. (Data taken from ISO 7029 [1984].)

the patient's family or friends than by the individual themselves. A patient will frequently complain of difficulties in understanding conversation in background noise and will often feel that others are not speaking clearly, rather than realising that it is their own hearing acuity that is changing. Over time, speech understanding declines more rapidly than the decline in the auditory thresholds.[3] Patients can begin to feel isolated because of communication difficulties, and there is a risk of depression. It is being increasingly recognised that hearing loss has a compounding effect on decline in mental function in dementia.

AETIOLOGY

Ageing affects all systems in the body, and the auditory system is no exception. 'Normal' hearing depends on a complicated interaction between the cochlea (the 'sensory' part of the system), the spiral ganglion neurons and the vestibulocochlear nerve (the 'neural' part of the system) and the central auditory pathway from vestibulocochlear nerve to the auditory cortex. Age-related changes will affect each part of the pathway to a different degree in each individual. In addition to the purely age-related changes, hearing may deteriorate due to exposure to environmental factors such as noise exposure (occupation- or recreational-related), ototoxic drugs and systemic diseases including diabetes and hypertension. The effects are seen at a cellular level in the cochlea, with a progressive decline in the number of outer and inner hair cells (**Figures 16.2A, B**), as well as changes in the stria vascularis, which affects homeostasis of the cochlear fluids. Apoptosis (programmed cell death) results in a decline in the number of cells throughout the auditory system, including spiral ganglion neurons and neurons in the central auditory pathway. It is not clear yet why it is the basal cochlear cells, which code for higher frequency sounds, that are most fragile, but they are also the ones most affected by these environmental factors.

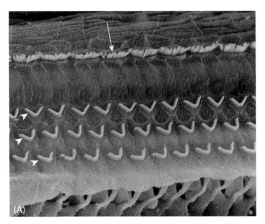 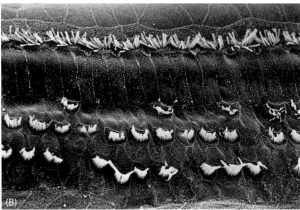

Figures 16.2A, B. Electron micrograph of normal outer (arrowheads) and inner (arrow) cochlear hair cells (16.2A). Electron micrograph of damaged hair cells in an aged cochlea (16.2B). (Images courtesy Marc Lenoir, from *Journey into the World of Hearing*, www.cochlea.org, by R Pujol *et al.*, NeurOreille, Montpellier.)

MANAGEMENT

Hearing aids are an effective means of providing auditory rehabilitation. However, no form of hearing aid will be able to restore hearing acuity back to normal, and patients can be frustrated that they still find it difficult to follow conversations in noisy situations. Management includes educating relatives in the use of clear speech. Where a severe to profound hearing loss is seen at high frequencies (thresholds over 80 dB at 2 and 4 kHz), cochlear implants are often more effective.

FUTURE DEVELOPMENTS

As research begins to clarify the specific changes that occur throughout the auditory system, novel drugs are being developed in an attempt to prevent, or reverse, damage at various points in the hearing pathway. Gene therapy may also have a role in regenerating new cochlear hair cells in due course. However, as there is no one single change that causes presbyacusis, it will be many years before there is an effective solution.

REFERENCES

1 MedlinePlus Medical Encyclopedia. http://nlm.nih.gov/medlineplus/ency/article/001045.htm
2 Chien W, Lin FR (2012) Prevalence of hearing aid use among older adults in the United States. *Arch Intern Med* **172(3):**292–293.
3 Divenyi PL, Stark PB, Haupt KM (2005) Decline of speech understanding and auditory thresholds in the elderly. *J Acoust Soc Am* **118(2):**1089–1100.

17

SUDDEN SENSORINEURAL HEARING LOSS

William P.L. Hellier

Contents

INTRODUCTION

Damage or change in the cochlear structures or the cochlear nerve leads to a sensorineural hearing loss (SNHL). A gradual SNHL over months or years is a common occurrence amongst the general population, usually caused by the ageing process leading to hair cell loss, but sometimes by other conditions. A sudden SNHL (SSNHL), occurring immediately or over a period of hours, is by comparison uncommon. It is usually defined as a 30 dB or greater SNHL in three contiguous frequencies that occurs over a period of less than 3 days.

The aetiology of SSNHL can be conveniently divided into traumatic and non-traumatic causes.

TRAUMATIC SUDDEN SENSORINEURAL HEARING LOSS

Traumatic SSNHL by its nature occurs immediately after an injury. The exact nature of the trauma is usually evident from the history.

▌ Direct trauma

Any object, such as a stick or a cotton bud, that is forced down the external ear canal may pierce the tympanic membrane (TM). Conductive hearing loss may occur due to damage to the TM or the ossicles, but if the stapes is subluxed or the round window membrane disrupted, a SSNHL can occur. Vertigo is more common if there has been a cochlear injury, and assessment with tuning forks in these cases is important, as a Weber test localising to the non-injured ear helps to differentiate a SNHL.

▌ Perilymph leak

Trauma can lead to disruption of either the stapes or the round window membrane. If this occurs, a leak of the perilymph from the inner ear will ensue. This will give a SNHL that can be sudden or potentially fluctuating. It is often associated with a fluctuating vertigo or imbalance. The most common cause is direct or indirect trauma, but a leak may occur with barotrauma (see below) or potentially raised intracranial pressure from straining or coughing. The last cause is unusual and there is some dispute about whether a true leak occurs in such cases.

▌ Post otologic surgery

Middle ear, stapes and mastoid surgery can lead to SSNHL. This can occur due to directly opening the inner ear either on purpose, as in stapedectomy or when removing cholesteatoma from an inner ear fistula, or inadvertently if the drill opens the lateral semicircular canal or is allowed to hit the ossicles. A profound SNHL may be evident postoperatively.

▌ Head injury and temporal bone fracture

Direct trauma to the skull can cause SSNHL either due to a fracture through the cochlea or because of shearing forces between the inner ear and neural structures. The petrous (Latin: rock) temporal bone is named because of its exceptionally hard and resistant nature. In order to fracture the temporal bone there usually has to be significant trauma, which will often lead to other neurological injuries and, almost undoubtedly, a period of loss of consciousness. Road traffic accidents are the most common cause (around 50%). Often a SSNHL due

to such trauma is overlooked initially because of the patient's other injuries. A CT scan of the temporal bone is the investigation of choice in such cases.

Temporal bone fractures are divided into longitudinal (down the axial axis of the temporal bone) and transverse fractures (across the axial axis). In reality, fractures are often a mix of the two types. Transverse fractures tend to cause SSNHL as they often extend across the cochlea and labyrinth (**Figure 17.1**), and balance disturbance is common. Longitudinal fractures more often involve the ossicles and middle ear (**Figure 17.2**) and lead to a conductive hearing loss. Tuning forks can help differentiate the difference in a bedside test. The facial nerve may be involved in either type of fracture.

SSNHL can occur with a head injury without a temporal bone fracture, when shearing forces across the cochlear nerve or cochlear structures lead to neural damage. A perilymph leak may also occur.

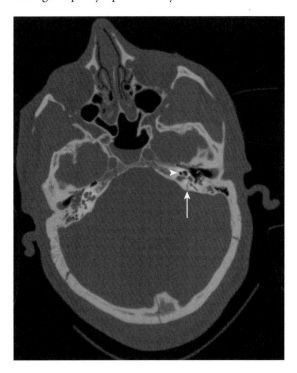

Figure 17.1. Transverse fracture of the temporal bone. Note the fracture line extending into the vestibule and cochlea (arrow) and the presence of air in the cochlea (arrowhead).

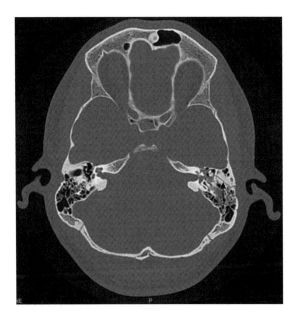

Figure 17.2. Longitudinal fracture of the temporal bone. Note the fracture (arrow) through the roof of the external canal to the area of the ossicles.

▌ Barotrauma

The pressure in the gas-filled space of the middle ear is regulated by the Eustachian tube. If the outer ear pressure changes rapidly and the middle ear does not 'equalize', then a mechanical pressure occurs across the eardrum due to the differential air pressure. This can be great enough to cause barotrauma to the ear. Barotrauma most commonly occurs when flying or diving. The greatest pressure change is in the first 10 metres of water submersion or the first 1,000 metres of air ascent, and if equalization does not occur, significant pressure can be generated across the TM. This more commonly causes middle ear changes such as bleeding or effusion, but if the pressure difference is marked between the middle ear and the cerebrospinal fluid/perilymph, a perilymph leak and SSNHL is possible.

SSNHL is also recognised in divers with decompression sickness. Too rapid an ascent from depth leads to gas bubbles forming in the blood and if these flow into the cochlear artery, they may cause vascular occlusion and cochlea hair cell death.

Explosions can cause barotrauma by way of a blast injury, significant energy being transferred to the inner ear, leading to membrane rupture and cell damage.

NON-TRAUMATIC HEARING LOSS

▌ Infective

Acute otitis media is a common condition and usually resolves without sequelae. However, bacterial toxins or frank infection can pass into the labyrinth, leading to SSNHL. Bacteria may also invade the cochlea from the cerebrospinal fluid, usually via the cochlear aqueduct, as is seen in meningitis. This causes hair cell death and can lead to ossification of the fluid-filled labyrinth. SSNHL is seen in 10% of patients with bacterial meningitis[1], and early referral for cochlear implantation is important where hearing loss is bilateral and profound, as cochlear ossification will prevent electrode insertion.

Viral infections have also been implicated in SSNHL. Ramsay Hunt syndrome occurs with herpes zoster infection, causing SNHL, facial nerve weakness, vesicles around the pinna and dizziness. Early recognition and treatment with anti-virals and steroids is beneficial, but many patients are left with some degree of SNHL.

▌ Idiopathic sudden sensorineural hearing loss

Idiopathic SSNHL describes the symptoms in a group of patients that have a sudden or rapidly evolving SNHL with no known cause. The definition of SSNHL in this case is usually taken as a 30 db or greater SNHL in three contiguous frequencies that occurs over less than 3 days.[2] Patients often wake with a feeling of blockage in one ear, but the hearing may deteriorate over a few days. They usually have a feeling of ear fullness or blockage and tinnitus, but no major balance symptoms. Often their hearing loss is thought to be, or diagnosed as, wax or middle ear fluid initially. Their presentation to an ENT department may occur late, when after some months the hearing has not returned. Assessment at the initial presentation with tuning forks is essential, as this will help differentiate a SNHL from a conductive hearing loss.

The incidence of idiopathic SSNHL is described as being between 8 and 20 cases per 100,000[2], and is reasonably commonly seen in ENT departments. A list of proposed causes of idiopathic SSNHL is shown in **Table 17.1** and a suggested set of investigations is given in **Table 17.2**.

Although hearing loss in SSNHL is defined as at least 30 dB, it is often greater and can be a complete hearing loss. Hearing improves in 50–65% of cases, usually in the first 1–3 weeks.[4,5] Improvement may be to the previous normal level, but many patients will be left with some residual SNHL. Poor prognostic features are severe to profound hearing loss and higher frequency losses.

The exact treatment of idiopathic SSNHL remains in doubt, partly because of its potentially heterogenous aetiology. As about 50% of cases will improve spontaneously, trials of therapy do not always yield a definite result. Many treatments have been used over the years including low molecular weight dextrans to increase blood flow and hyperbaric oxygen.

Table 17.1. Proposed causes of idiopathic sudden sensorineural hearing loss.

Cause	Mechanism
Vascular	Occlusion of cochlear vessels or vascular spasm
Viral infection	Viral cochlea inflammation similar to viral vestibulitis
Vestibular schwannoma	Tumour growth causing vascular compromise[3]
Autoimmune	Specific antibody damage to cochlear structures or as part of more general autoimmune disease
Hyperviscosity syndromes	Vascular compromise of cochlear blood flow
Multiple sclerosis	Change of neural transmission

Table 17.2. Suggested investigations for idiopathic sudden sensorineural hearing loss.

Investigation	Reason
Full blood count	Exclude high haemoglobin or systemic disorder
ESR and CRP	Exclude inflammatory/autoimmune cause
Autoantibodies	Look for autoimmune cause
Cholesterol and lipid profile	Look for risk factors for vascular occlusion
Syphilis serology	Rarely, syphilis can cause SSNHL
Glucose level	Exclude diabetes
MRI of IAM	Exclude acoustic neuroma/look for vascular disease and demyelination

ESR, erythrocyte sedimentation rate; CRP, C-reactive protein; IAM, internal auditory meatus.

Table 17.3. Treatment of idiopathic sudden sensorineural hearing loss.

Treatment	Rationale
Oral corticosteroids (prednisolone 40–60 mg once daily for 1 week)	To reduce any inflammatory cause
Antiviral medication (acyclovir 200–400 mg 5 times daily for 7 days)	To treat any viral cause
Betahistine (16 mg three times daily for 4 weeks)	To improve cochlear blood flow
Inhaled carbogen (5% CO_2, 95% O_2) 5 minutes every hour for 24 hours if the patient presents within a week of the sudden sensorineural hearing loss	To improve cochlear blood flow by cerebral vasodilatation

No single therapy has been shown to be truly effective, but most departments and ENT surgeons have come to a pragmatic treatment regimen, which looks to give the most potential help, while being relatively easy to administer and avoid major side-effects. The author's personal and departmental practice is to give the medications listed in **Table 17.3** if the patient presents in the first 2–3 weeks after the onset of the idiopathic SSNHL. There is no good evidence that drug therapy can influence the outcome if commenced 3–4 weeks post hearing loss.

There is some evidence that intratympanic injection of steroids may lead to hearing improvement with fewer side-effects than the systemic administration of steroids. However, trials as discussed above are inconclusive, and further research is needed.

REFERENCES

1 Baraff LJ, Lee SI, Schriger DL (1993) Outcomes of bacterial meningitis in children: a meta-analysis. *Pediatr Infect Dis J* **12**:389–394.

2 Hughes G, Freedman M, Haberkamp T (1996) Sudden sensorineural hearing loss. *Otolaryngol Clin North Am* **29**:393–405.

3 Moffat DA Baguley DM, von Blumenthal H *et al.* (1994) Sudden deafness in vestibular schwannoma. *J Laryngol Otol* **108**:116–119.

4 Mattox D, Simmons F (1977) Natural history of sudden sensorineural hearing loss. *Ann Otol Rhinol Laryngol* **86**:463–480.

5 Wilson WR, Byl FM, Laird N (1980) The efficacy of steroids in the treatment of idiopathic sudden hearing loss. A double blind clinical study. *Arch Otolaryngol* **106**:772–776.

18

NOISE-INDUCED HEARING LOSS

Stephen Broomfield

Contents

INTRODUCTION

Noise-induced hearing loss (NIHL) can be reversible (temporary threshold shift), with recovery in hours to days, or permanent (permanent threshold shift). Permanent NIHL most commonly follows repeated noise exposure over a long period of time, but can occur following a single loud noise exposure, known as acoustic trauma. Noise that is sufficiently loud to cause injury can broadly be categorised as occupational, environmental or recreational (**Table 18.1**). NIHL is a significant worldwide health burden, a major cause of avoidable hearing impairment and a leading cause of occupational compensation.[1]

MECHANISM

While the exact mechanism of NIHL is incompletely understood, it is well recognised that in most cases NIHL is multifactorial, with a complex interaction between genetic and environmental factors. Cochlear damage is likely to be due to a combination of metabolic disturbance, oxidative stress and physical injury, with outer hair cells most commonly affected in the early stages. Predisposing factors include smoking, diabetes and ototoxic agents. Neonates, the elderly and low socio-economic groups may also be more susceptible.[2] There is commonly an overlap with age-related or idiopathic sensorineural hearing loss.

Table 18.1. Common potential causes of noise-induced hearing loss.

Occupational	Environmental	Recreational
Military	Road traffic	Bars, nightclubs
Aircraft	Air traffic	Personal music players
Engineering/construction	Railways	Concerts
Factories	Construction	Mobile phones
Music industry		Sports (e.g. motor sports)
Call centres		

PRESENTATION/DIAGNOSIS

Patients may present with hearing loss or be picked up as part of an occupational screening programme. Initially, difficulty hearing in background noise is common, leading to a loss of clarity (e.g. with the television or telephone). Tinnitus and hyperacusis are also common and their onset related to noise exposure supports the diagnosis of NIHL. Patients experiencing acoustic trauma may describe otalgia or dizziness. As the hearing loss progresses, symptoms may become more disruptive, ultimately leading to loss of social interaction, reduced confidence and mood disturbance. Ascertaining a detailed history of noise exposure is critical. The level and duration of the noise exposure are important, as well as use of ear protection.

A pure tone audiogram is the most important investigation and will classically show a dip in high frequency sensory thresholds at 4 or 6 KHz (**Figure 18.1**).

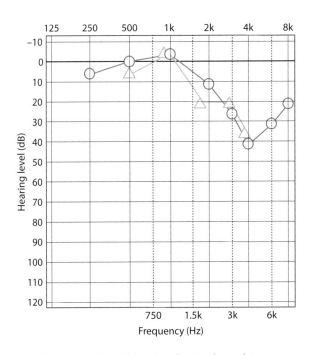

Figure 18.1. Audiogram showing noise-induced hearing loss in the right ear.

This typical pattern may not be seen clearly in patients with co-existing presbyacusis. Significant asymmetry is uncommon, although may be seen in cases where rifle shooting is a contributing factor; in such cases the ear furthest from the rifle's barrel is protected from the gunfire noise by the shadow effect of the head. Recently, there has been interest in the use of otoacoustic emissions in the screening and diagnosis of NIHL.[3]

NOISE-INDUCED HEARING LOSS AND THE LAW

NIHL remains a common cause of medico-legal claims. A successful claim relies on separating out co-existent inner ear pathologies from NIHL. In particular, allowing for age-related hearing loss is challenging. Tables and formulae to adjust for average age-related hearing thresholds in the population exist for this purpose and estimate the disability associated with a particular hearing loss.[4] In the UK, some occupations may be eligible to claim social benefits for NIHL from the Industrial Injuries Disablement Benefit or the Armed Forces Compensation Scheme.

In order to protect workers and reduce the cost of claims, specific laws concerning NIHL have developed. In the UK, the Health and Safety Executive 'Control of Noise at Work Regulations 2005'[5] govern the law in this area, and contain rules on maximum permitted sound pressure levels as well as formulae for calculating an employee's daily and weekly personal noise exposure levels based on the noise level and duration of exposure. These limits determine what measures an employer must take to protect the employee (summarised in **Table 18.2**).

In the NIHL field, sound pressure levels are most commonly described using the A-weighted decibel scale, which accounts for the relative loudness of low level sounds perceived by the human ear at different frequencies. The C-weighted scale follows the frequency sensitivity of the human ear at very high noise levels by including more of the low frequency range of sounds; it is used to describe noise levels thought to be potentially damaging.

Table 18.2. Noise levels and measures required by employers under UK law.

Daily or weekly PNE	Peak SPL	Measures required
80 dBA	135 dBC	Adjust machinery, fit silencers, enclose in separate room Minimise duration of exposure to noise for each employee Regular hearing tests/surveillance Provision and maintenance of ear protection Education and training of employees
85 dBA	137 dBC	As above – but use of ear protection mandatory
87 dBA	140 dBC	Maximum permitted levels (with hearing protection)

PNE, personal noise exposure; SPL, sound pressure level; dBA/dBC, A-weighted and C-weighted decibel scales (for description see text).

TREATMENT AND PREVENTION

Prevention of NIHL requires effective education regarding the risks of noise to hearing. While changes in the law have limited occupational NIHL in developed countries, there is still a lot of work to be done in the developing world. The effectiveness of hearing protection devices depends on training and proper use, and stricter legislation is therefore unlikely to reduce NIHL in the absence of wider educational programmes.[6] Similarly, increasing use of personal music players in young people cannot be legislated for and may lead to a rise in NIHL cases in future.

For people with established NIHL, treatment is largely supportive. Provision of hearing aids may be indicated for some, and therapy for tinnitus or hyperacusis may also be necessary.

FUTURE TREATMENTS

As the understanding of the mechanism of NIHL improves, promising new treatments are emerging. There has been considerable interest in the use of otoprotective agents, including dietary and pharmacologic anti-oxidants. Results of clinical trials in the military are awaited.[7] Research examining the genetic factors predisposing to NIHL may allow for targeted population screening and prophylactic use of new medications. Advances in inner ear biological research also bring the potential for hearing improvements through hair cell regeneration using gene therapy and stem cell therapy.[8]

REFERENCES

1 World Health Organisation (1997) *Prevention of Noise-induced Hearing Loss. Report of an Informal Consultation held at the WHO*. World Health Organisation, Geneva.

2 van Kamp I, Davies H (2013) Noise and health in vulnerable groups. *Noise Health* **15:**153–159.

3 Basner M, Babisch W, Davis A *et al.* (2014) Auditory and non-auditory effects of noise on health. *Lancet* **383:**1325–1332.

4 International Organisation for Standardization (ISO) (1999:2013). *Acoustics. Estimation of Noise-Induced Hearing Loss*, 3rd edn. International Organisation for Standardization, Geneva.

5 Health and Safety Executive (2005) *Control of Noise at Work Regulations, 2005*. HMSO, London.

6 Verbeek JH, Kateman E, Morata TC *et al.* (2012) Interventions to prevent occupational noise-induced hearing loss. *Cochrane Database Syst Revs* Issue 10, Art. No. CD006396. doi: 10.1002/14651858.CD006396.pub3.

7 Slowinska-Kowalska M, Davis A (2012) Noise-induced hearing loss. *Noise Health* **14:**274–280.

8 Rubel EW, Furrer SA, Stone JS (2013) A brief history of hair cell regeneration research and speculations on the future. *Hearing Res* **297:**42–51.

19

AUTOIMMUNE INNER EAR HEARING LOSS

Bruno Kenway & James R. Tysome

Contents

DEFINITION

Autoimmune-related hearing loss, described by McCabe in 1979[1], is characterized by a rapidly progressing, usually bilateral hearing loss, which may fluctuate over a period of weeks to months. The duration and pattern distinguishes this condition from the more gradual hearing loss seen in presbyacusis and the abrupt loss in sudden sensorineural hearing loss. Responsiveness to steroid or immunosuppressant treatment is also considered characteristic of autoimmune inner ear disease (AIED). Vestibular symptoms are common and accompany up to 50% of cases.

EPIDEMIOLOGY

AIED is likely to represent only 1% of cases of hearing loss, although this may be an underestimate. It usually affects those between the ages of 30 and 60, and is more common in females.

CAUSES

AIED is divided into patients where only the inner ear is affected (primary AIED) and those cases caused by systemic autoimmune conditions (approximately 20% of cases). There are various theories as to the mechanism by which autoimmune conditions may cause hearing loss: antibodies may cause accidental inner ear damage due to the presence of antigens shared by the ear and the intended target of the antibody (so called 'molecular mimicry'); release of cytokines by the damaged inner ear may evoke delayed immune reactions (known as Bystander damage). Some systemic autoimmune conditions, such as Wegener's granulomatosis and Churg–Strauss syndrome, can also cause conductive hearing loss through middle ear disease. AIED should also be considered in patients with Ménière's disease affecting one ear who subsequently develop fluctuating hearing thresholds in the contralateral ear. The differential diagnosis also includes perilymph fistula and sudden sensorineural hearing loss.

PRIMARY AUTOIMMUNE INNER EAR DISEASE (THE INNER EAR AS THE SINGLE AFFECTED ORGAN)

The key factors indicative of AIED are summarised in **Table 19.1**. Arriving at a diagnosis of AIED can be challenging, particularly when there is no suggestion of systemic autoimmune disease. Currently, the OtoBlot test represents a commercially available western blot assay for anti-heat shock protein 70 (HSP) antibodies. This was previously known as the 68-kd protein antibody and is positive in 5% of the normal population. The sensitivity and specificity of this test are 42% and 90%, respectively, with a positive predictive value of 91%.[2] In primary AIED, antibodies to HSP 70 have also been identified in up to 47% of Ménière's disease patients, suggesting a possible immunological role for the disease. Twenty-five percent of AIED patients have raised inner ear specific IFN-γ-producing T cells.[3] While a positive test for HSP 70 may predict whether the patient is responsive to steroids and can therefore be used clinically to guide treatment[4], it is not widely available and the clinical picture is primarily used to make a diagnosis.

Table 19.1. Summary of key features for diagnosis of autoimmune inner ear disease.

● Sensorineural hearing loss of 30 dB or more at any frequency with evidence of progression on serial audiograms less than 3 months apart
● Normal MRI in asymmetric cases
● Laboratory tests suggestive of systemic autoimmune disease or single organ AIED
● Positive response to steroid treatment

SYSTEMIC AUTOIMMUNE CONDITIONS

The most frequently encountered systemic auto-immune conditions affecting hearing will now be outlined. The tests to try to confirm their presence are listed in **Table 19.2**. This is not an exhaustive account and other conditions include Goodpasture syndrome, myasthenia gravis, Behcet's disease, Sjogren's, antiphospholipid syndrome and Lyme's disease.

▮ Wegener's granulomatosis (now called granulomatosis with polyangiitis)

This necrotising granulomatous vasculitis affects the respiratory tract and kidneys. Over half of patients with Wegener's have hearing loss, of which half are sensorineural.[5] The hearing loss often precedes the formal diagnosis of Wegener's and the otolaryngologist should be mindful of this. C-antineutrophil cytoplasmic antibody positivity strongly supports the diagnosis. In common with other systemic causes, the mechanism of action is thought to be vasculitis of the cochlear arteries.

▮ Relapsing polychondritis

Twenty percent of affected individuals may have sensorineural hearing loss and it has been proposed that vasculitis of the labyrinthine artery is the causative factor. It is characterised by cartilage inflammation and destruction, usually of the pinna with sparing of the earlobe. Tracheal involvement can also occur and antibodies to type 2 collagen are frequently found. There are no diagnostic laboratory tests available but a raised erythrocyte sedimention rate or C-reactive protein is supportive and cartilage biopsy will show chondrolysis, chondritis and perichondritis.

▮ Cogan's syndrome

Cogan's syndrome is a rare autoimmune vasculitis characterised by ocular symptoms (typically interstitial keratitis) and audiovestibular problems that can mimic Ménière's disease. The diagnosis is made purely on clinical suspicion, although syphilis can present similarly and should be excluded.

▮ Polyarteritis nodosa

This medium-vessel vasculitis can cause rapid onset sensorineural hearing loss, often associated with facial nerve palsy. Systemic features include abdominal pain, myalgia and skin rashes.

Table 19.2. Diagnostic tests for common systemic autoimmune conditions.

Condition	Diagnostic tests
Wegener's granulomatosis	C-antineutrophil cytoplasmic antibodies
Cogan's syndrome	Clinical diagnosis, exclude syphilis
Relapsing polychondritis	Erythrocyte sedimentation rate, C-reactive protein, consider cartilage biopsy
Systemic lupus erythematosus	Anti-DS DNA, antinuclear antibody, antiphospholipid antibody
Polyarteritis nodosa	Myeloperoxidase antineutrophil cytoplasmic antibodies
Sarcoidosis	Angiotensin-converting enzyme

▌ Systemic lupus erythematosus

While it has been proposed that sensorineural hearing loss is more common in subjects with systemic lupus erythematosus, this is not universally accepted.[6] Multi-organ involvement is typical, with malar rash, discoid rash and arthropathy common.

▌ Sarcoidosis

Sarcoidosis is a multi-organ disease characterised by non-caseating granulomata. Classical features include arthralgia, bilateral hilar lymphadenopathy and erythema nodosum. Colvin[7] reviewed cases of audiovestibular manifestations of sarcoidosis in the medical literature and concluded that the likely cause was vestibulocochlear nerve neuropathy.

TREATMENT

In systemic cases of secondary AIED with hearing loss, the patient is best managed in a multidisciplinary manner with rheumatologists, otolaryngologists and audiologists. Immunosuppression is the mainstay of treatment for primary single organ AIED.

Rauch *et al.*[8] have proposed a high-dose prednisolone regime of 1 mg/kg/day for 4 weeks. Steroid responders should continue treatment until audiograms stabilise, before tapering the dose.

Intratympanic steroid treatment may be beneficial in refractory cases and has been shown to improve hearing loss and vestibular symptoms in small studies.[9] A treatment protocol is outlined in **Figure 19.1**. In patients unable to tolerate steroids, alternative immune modulating treatments have been used including cyclophosphamide, methotrexate and rituximab; these require specialist monitoring, generally by rheumatologists. Plasmapheresis has also been investigated as a treatment option, although the role of this remains uncertain.[10]

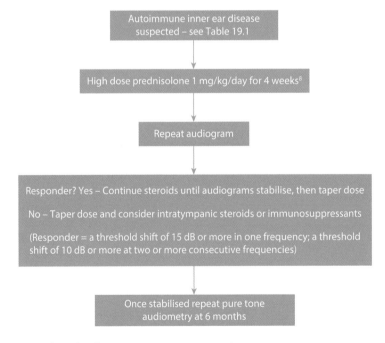

Figure 19.1. Treatment algorithm for autoimmune inner ear disease.

CONCLUSIONS

Clinicians need a high index of suspicion in order to diagnose AIED. Progressive bilateral hearing loss should trigger careful evaluation to exclude systemic autoimmune conditions. Glucocorticoids represent the mainstay of treatment.

REFERENCES

1 McCabe BF (1979) Autoimmune sensorineural hearing loss. *Ann Otol Rhinol Laryngol* **88(5 Pt 1):**585–589.
2 Hirose K, Wener MH, Duckert LG (1999) Utility of laboratory testing in autoimmune inner ear disease. *Laryngoscope* **109:**1749–1754.
3 Lorenz RR, Solares CA, Williams P *et al.* (2002) Interferon-gamma production to inner ear antgensby T cells from patients with autoimmune sensorineural hearing loss. *J Neuroimmunol* **130:**173–178.
4 Moscicki RA, San Martin JE, Quintero CH *et al.* (1994) Serum antibody to inner ear proteins in patients with progressive hearing loss. Correlation with disease activity and response to corticosteroid treatment. *J Am Med Assoc* **272:**611–616.
5 Bakthavachalam S, Driver MS, Cox C *et al.* (2004) Hearing loss in Wegener's granulomatosis. *Otol Neurotol* **25(5):**833–837.
6 Kastanioudakis I, Ziavra N, Voulgari PV *et al.* (2002) Ear involvement in systemic lupus erythematosus patients: a comparative study. *J Laryngol Otol* **116(2):**103–107.
7 Colvin IB (2006) Audiovestibular manifestations of sarcoidosis: a review of the literature. *Laryngoscope* **116(1):**75–82.
8 Rauch SD (1997) Clinical management of immune-mediated inner ear disease. *Ann NY Acad Sci* **830:**203–210.
9 Harris DA, Mkikulec AA, Carls SL (2013) Autoimmune inner ear disease preliminary case report: audiometric findings following steroid treatments. *Am J Audiol* **22(1):**120–124.
10 Luetje CM, Berliner KI (1997) Plasmapheresis in autoimmune inner ear disease: long-term follow-up. *Am J Otol* **18:**572–576.

20
COCHLEAR IMPLANTATION

Maarten de Wolf & Richard Irving

Contents

INTRODUCTION

Cochlear implantation represents one of the greatest medical advances of the 20th century and hearing remains the only one of the senses that can be medically restored to something approaching its original form. Cochlear implants (CIs) are indicated for patients with severe to profound sensorineural hearing loss where conventional acoustic amplification is not beneficial. They are placed in the cochlea and stimulate the auditory nerve directly. CIs are proven to be cost effective[1]; however, it is suspected that only a small proportion of potential adult CI candidates have received one.

ELECTRICAL STIMULATION OF THE AUDITORY SYSTEM

CIs use the tonotopic organisation of the auditory nerve fibres to provide frequency specific stimulation. They consist of an internal and an external component.

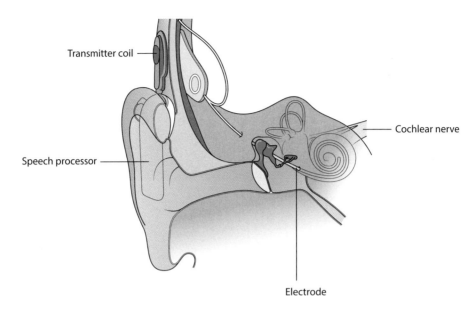

Transmitter coil

Cochlear nerve

Speech processor

Electrode

Figure 20.1. Cochlear implant: external and internal components.

The external component includes a microphone, speech processor, power source and radiofrequency transmitter. The device is worn behind the ear and held over the internal device by a magnet (**Figure 20.1**). The speech processor filters the acoustic signal and transforms it into an electric signal.

The internal component consists of an electrode array coupled to a hermetically sealed electronics package, a telemetry coil and a magnet, and transfers the electric signal to the cochlear nerve.

INDICATIONS

In the UK, National Institute for Clinical Excellence (NICE)[1] guidelines state that adults are eligible for cochlear implantation after having had at least 3 months of aided hearing, if their unaided hearing level is 90 dB or worse at frequencies 2 and 4 kHz and if their aided speech discrimination score is 50% or less at a sound intensity of 70 dB SPL.

In children, the same unaided hearing levels apply with emphasis on the child's sound awareness and delay in speech and language development. Simultaneous bilateral implantation is available for all children and visually impaired adults.

CANDIDATE ASSESSMENT

▌ Adults

A multidisciplinary assessment should be carried out with particular emphasis on the history related to the

loss of hearing. Better outcomes are typically achieved with a shorter duration of deafness and in those with a current or recent history of hearing aid use. Realistic expectations of outcome need to be discussed.

The selection of which ear to implant can prove difficult. The ear with better speech recognition leads to the best audiometric result. On the other hand, however, patients do best with bimodal hearing and may want to keep a hearing aid that is still giving them some benefit.

▌ Children

To achieve the best possible outcomes in pre-lingually deaf children, it is now widely accepted to implant at the youngest age possible. Implantation before the age of 2 years is more likely to result in nearly normal hearing development.

The recommended bilateral placement of CIs significantly improves hearing in noisy environments and allows for the ability to localise sound. Simultaneous placement increases the chances for binaural hearing.[2]

IMAGING

Preoperative MRI is used to demonstrate the status of the cochlear nerve, pathology in the cerebellopontine angle and malformations of the cochlea.

CT is used to demonstrate bony anatomy and malformations of the inner ear.

SURGERY

The aim of cochlear implantation is to place an electrode in the cochlea close to the cochlear nerve endings. Usually, a CI is placed via a retro-auricular incision exposing the mastoid while creating sufficient access to the soft tissue to place the processor in a well drilled into the skull. Access to the cochlea is achieved by cortical mastoidectomy and a posterior tympanotomy to open the facial recess. The electrode is placed into the scala tympani, either through the round window membrane or via a separate cochleostomy (**Figure 20.2**).

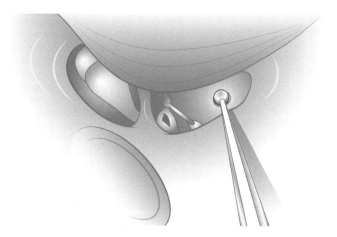

Figure 20.2. Through the posterior tympanotomy, access to the scala tympani of the cochlea is achieved either by performing a cochleostomy or by exposing the round window membrane.

▌ Complications

Complications after implantation are uncommon. Medical problems include wound infection and delayed healing, taste disturbance, imbalance and facial weakness. Device-related complications include hard failures, such as dysfunction of the internal device, and soft failures such as pain, shocking sensations, atypical tinnitus, facial nerve stimulation and diminishing function.

SURGICAL SPECIAL CONSIDERATIONS

In approximately 20% of children undergoing cochlear implantation, congenital inner ear malformations are present. These include common cavity deformity, cerebrospinal fluid gushers (**Figure 20.3**), hypoplastic cochlea, absent semicircular canals, external auditory canal atresia and cochlear nerve deficiency. These findings pose an extra challenge for cochlea implantation and should be managed with extra care.

Cochlear obstruction can occur after trauma and meningitis. In the latter, cochlear implantation should be performed as soon as possible, as cochlear ossification and fibrosis may occur soon after meningitis and prevent insertion of the CI electrode (**Figures 20.4A, B**).

EXTENDED INDICATIONS

Congenitally deafened adults are now increasingly coming forward for implantation. Although in many benefit is restricted to improvements in environmental sound perception, this can be hugely advantageous. Those with no discernable speech or no history of hearing aid use should be discouraged.

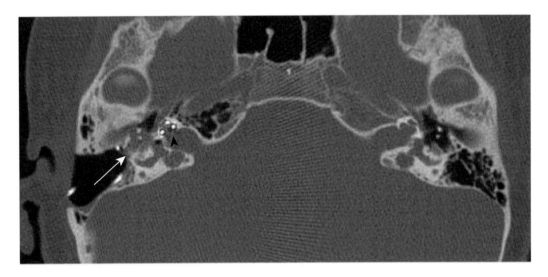

Figure 20.3. Inner ear malformation in X-linked stapes gusher. The lateral end of the internal auditory meatus communicates directly with the cochlear lumen. A right side cochlear implant (black arrowhead) and soft tissue plug (white arrow) used to seal the cerebrospinal fluid leak.

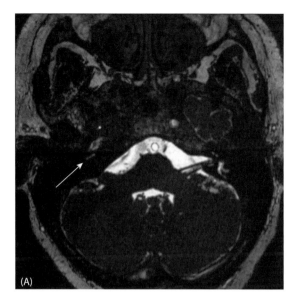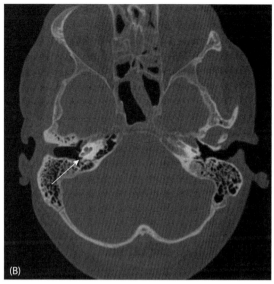

Figures 20.4A, B. CT image and MRI scan demonstrating partial obliteration of the cochlear lumen. The MRI scan demonstrates little normal signal from the cochlea (arrow) and the CT image shows some evidence of new bone formation in the basal turn (arrow).

Sadly, bilateral CIs are still not accepted as standard treatment in adults, although they are beneficial for speech perception in noise under certain conditions.

CIs are also not yet a standard treatment for single sided deafness in adults or children, despite increasing evidence to support their benefits.[3]

OUTCOMES

The ultimate goal of hearing rehabilitation is to enable understanding of speech in everyday environments; this, however, is not a realistic aim for all.

Several factors influence the level of performance. These include the aetiology of the hearing loss, the level of residual hearing, cochlear anatomy and nerve status, the mode of communication and access to good rehabilitation.

Improved outcome is associated with surgical factors such as an atraumatic technique, slow electrode insertion, round window insertion and the use of perioperative steroids.

FUTURE

Cochlear implantation is in many respects the ultimate alliance between medicine and technology and it continues to evolve in line with advances in both these areas. Developments might be seen in auditory processing aiming at environmental and music appreciation, shifting of implantation criteria to patients with asymmetric and single sided losses, robotic aided surgery, single unit external processors and miniaturisation of hardware and totally implantable devices.

Hearing loss is the most frequent sensory deficit that afflicts mankind, with 80% of the population with hearing loss residing in the low and medium income countries. Many of these individuals do not have access to cochlear implants, and the biggest advance imaginable would be to extend access worldwide to all who could potentially benefit.

REFERENCES

1 National Institute for Health and Care Excellence (2009) NICE Tchnology appraisal guidance (TA 166). Cochlear implants for children and adults with severe to profound deafness [Internet]. Cochlear implants for children and adults with severe to profound deafness. [cited 2014 Sep 21]. Available from: http://www.nice.org.uk/guidance/ta166#.VB8kEMJhUN4.mendeley.

2 Ramsden JD, Gordon K, Aschendorff A *et al.* (2012) European Bilateral Pediatric Cochlear Implant Forum consensus statement. *Otol Neurotol* **33(4):**561–565. Available from: http://www.ncbi.nlm.nih.gov/pubmed/22569146.

3 Van Schoonhoven J, Sparreboom M, van Zanten BG *et al.* (2013) The effectiveness of bilateral cochlear implants for severe-to-profound deafness in adults: a systematic review. *Otol Neurotol* **34(2):**190–198. Available from: http://www.ncbi.nlm.nih.gov/pubmed/2344446.

21

TUMOURS OF THE CEREBELLOPONTINE ANGLE

Patrick Axon

Contents

INTRODUCTION

Tumours of the cerebellopontine angle are rare, invariably benign and slow growing. Vestibular schwannomas are by far the commonest of these tumours and as the name implies, arise from the myelin sheath of the vestibular nerve within the internal auditory meatus. As these tumours grow, they expand into the cerebellopontine angle, which is the cerebrospinal fluid space separating the petrous temporal bone from the brain (**Figure 21.1**). If a growing vestibular schwannoma is left unchecked, it progressively compresses the brainstem, eventually causing patient death.

CLINICAL PRESENTATION/SYMPTOMS

Patients usually present with unilateral hearing loss often associated with imbalance and ipsilateral tinnitus. Rarely, patients will also complain of ear discomfort, facial twitch and ipsilateral facial numbness or paraesthesia as a result of compression of the trigeminal nerve. Early symptoms are often well tolerated by patients, resulting in many years of delay before seeking advice. If a patient presents with unilateral hearing loss of over 6 weeks' duration, then referral to an ENT specialist is advised.

Patient examination is often normal other than tuning fork tests demonstrating a sensorineural hearing loss and some unsteadiness on balance testing. Pure tone audiometry will demonstrate an asymmetric sensorineural hearing loss predominantly affecting the higher frequencies. Skull base units offering specialised patient care will also perform speech discrimination tests to help guide patients in their future management decisions.

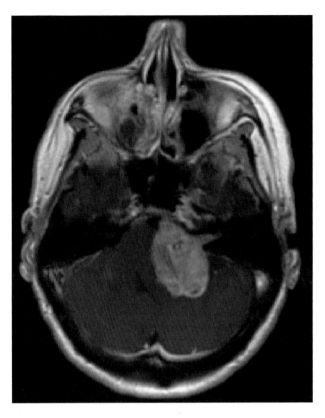

Figure 21.1. Large left vestibular schwannoma causing brainstem compression.

PATHOGENESIS

Hearing loss is caused by a combination of pressure on the auditory nerve and loss of cochlear function. These two causes of hearing loss result in different types of hearing disability. Progressive loss of cochlear function will primarily cause a rise in hearing thresholds but with speech understanding usually well maintained. In this situation, well-fitted hearing aids may deliver significant patient benefit. However, progressive loss of auditory nerve function will result in substantial loss of speech understanding, making hearing aids far less effective. This makes speech discrimination tests invaluable for assessing whether a patient would benefit from a hearing aid.

INVESTIGATION

Around 7% of patients presenting with an asymmetric sensorineural hearing loss (15 dB hearing loss or greater at 2 or more frequencies) have a vestibular schwannoma.[1] All patients with a significant asymmetry should therefore undergo MR imaging, as should any patient with unilateral tinnitus.

MANAGEMENT

The management of patients with a vestibular schwannoma is dependent on patient preference, tumour size, patient age and patient symptoms. A detailed description of treatment algorithms is beyond the scope of this chapter, but if a tumour has an intracranial tumour diameter of >30 mm, surgery will usually be the treatment of choice. Patients with smaller tumours have a choice of management options including tumour surveillance with serial MRI, surgery and radiotherapy (stereotactic radiosurgery [SRS] for small tumours and fractionated radiotherapy for larger tumours). Specialist skull base units will offer all forms of treatment and present the patient with the relative risks and benefits of each to allow them to make a decision.

Many patients with small tumours will opt for tumour surveillance. It is estimated that only 30% of small tumours will grow over the subsequent 5 years, so a large proportion of patients who have stable tumours will also have useful ipsilateral hearing.[2] A large proportion of patients will have poor ipsilateral hearing at presentation and aiding might increase distortion and, paradoxically, make overall hearing worse. Patients who do not have useful hearing in their tumour ear might benefit from a CROS (Contralateral Routing of Sound) aid. The transmitter is placed behind or inside the poorer hearing ear. This picks up sound and transmits it wirelessly to a receiver in the normal hearing ear. In patients with a degree of hearing loss in the non-tumour ear, the BiCROS (Bilateral CROS) aid transmits sound to a hearing aid that also serves as an amplifier, improving hearing in that ear. An alternative method is the bone-anchored hearing aid (see Chapter 14: Bone-anchored hearing aids), which when implanted on the tumour side, transmits sound directly to the contralateral normal hearing cochlea as vibrations across the bones of the skull. This technique means that patients do not have to wear two hearing aid devices and for some patients this is more acceptable.

Some units advocate active treatment for small tumours arguing that early intervention offers a probability of maintaining residual useful hearing and tumour control.[3] Kano et al.[4] demonstrated 89% long-term maintenance of good hearing following SRS. Woodson et al.[5] demonstrated 78% good long-term hearing preservation after middle fossa resection of small tumours. However, it should be remembered that 70% of these small tumours will not grow long term and that 87% of patients with good hearing will maintain their good hearing long term with no intervention.[6] Patients should therefore be enabled to make an informed treatment decision incorporating all hearing technologies.

REFERENCES

1 Cueva RA (2004) Auditory brainstem response versus magnetic resonance imaging for the evaluation of asymmetric sensorineural hearing loss. *Laryngoscope* **114(10)**:1686–1692.

2 Hughes M, Skilbeck C, Saeed S et al. (2011) Expectant management of vestibular schwannoma: a retrospective multivariate analysis of tumor growth and outcome. *Skull Base* **21(5)**:295–302.

3 Kano H, Kondziolka D, Khan A et al. (2013) Predictors of hearing preservation after stereotactic radiosurgery for acoustic neuroma: clinical article. *J Neurosurg* **119(Suppl)**:863–873.

4 Woodson EA1, Dempewolf RD, Gubbels SP et al. (2010) Long-term hearing preservation after microsurgical excision of vestibular schwannoma. *Otol Neurotol* **31(7)**:1144–1152.

5 Eljamel S, Hussain M, Eljamel MS (2011) Should initial surveillance of vestibular schwannoma be abandoned? *Skull Base* **21(1)**:59–64.

6 Stangerup SE, Thomsen J, Tos M et al. (2010) Long-term hearing preservation in vestibular schwannoma. *Otol Neurotol* **31(2)**:271–275.

22 OTOTOXICITY

Aaron Trinidade & James R. Tysome

Contents

INTRODUCTION

Ototoxicity is defined as injury to the function of the inner ear caused by a drug. The term is used to broadly describe injury of both hearing and balance, although drugs may be more specifically termed cochleotoxic or vestibulotoxic depending on the part of the inner ear they preferentially affect.

The drugs most commonly attributed to causing ototoxicity include aminoglycosides, platinum-based chemotherapeutic agents, salicylates, loop diuretics and quinines. Ototoxicity typically results in high frequency sensorineural hearing loss (SNHL), tinnitus and, if the vestibular system is also affected, imbalance. Symptoms may vary depending on the mechanism of action of the ototoxic drug. Hearing loss may affect both ears and is often irreversible (**Table 22.1**). The onset of symptoms is also variable, ranging from within days to weeks or months following completion of the drug administration. The most common groups of ototoxic drugs will be described.

AMINOGLYCOSIDES

Aminoglycosides are the most common class of drugs causing ototoxicity. They include streptomycin, dihydrostreptomycin, kanamycin, gentamicin, tobramycin, netilmicin and amikacin, with neomycin the most cochleotoxic. The true incidence of ototoxicity amongst these drugs is

Table 22.1. Summary of the main ototoxic drugs and their effects.

Drug	Effect on inner ear	Clinical effects	Reversible	Dose-dependent	Risk factors
Aminoglycosides			No	Yes	Genetic predisposition
Dihydrostreptomycin Amikacin Neomycin Kanamicin	Cochleotoxic: apoptosis of OHCs, especially basal turn of cochlea	High frequency SNHL			
Streptomycin Tobramycin Netlimicin	Vestibulotoxic: apoptosis of Type1 >Type 2 hair cells of vestibular system	Imbalance, oscillopsia			
Gentamicin	Vestibulocochleotoxic	Tinnitus, high frequency SNHL and vertigo			
Loop diuretics	Vestibulocochleotoxic: alteration of the striae vascularis ion exchange systems between causing gradient changes between endolymph and perilymph	Tinnitus and dysequilibrium	Yes	Yes	Renal failure
Platinum-based chemotherapeutics	Cochleotoxic: free-radical generation within the striae vascularis causing apoptosis of OHCs, especially basal turn of cochlea	Tinnitus, and high frequency SNHL	No	Yes	Renal failure
Salicylates	Cochleotoxic: multifactorial effects on spiral ganglion neurons	Tinnitus and high frequency SNHL	Yes	Yes	Advanced age; dehydration

OHC, outer hair cells; SNHL, sensorineural hearing loss.

unknown but is thought to be underestimated and may be as high as 47% when ultra-high frequencies (>8 kHz) are considered. These drugs vary in their differential effect on the vestibulocochlear system, with dihydrostreptomycin, amikacin, neomycin and kanamycin being more cochleotoxic, and streptomycin, tobramycin and netlimicin more vestibulotoxic. Gentamicin may affect both systems, but is thought to be primarily vestibulotoxic, hence its use as an intratympanic injection to ablate the vestibular system in Ménière's disease.

Aminoglycosides affect the outer hair cells (OHCs) of the organ of Corti, primarily at the basal turn of the cochlea, resulting in the typical high frequency SNHL (frequencies >4 kHz are affected first), and primarily the Type 1 hair cells of the vestibular system, causing imbalance and nystagmus, which can progress to oscillopsia. Aminoglycoside ototoxicity is usually permanent. The exact mechanism of how this injury occurs is unknown but is thought to be due to the generation of free radicals within the inner ear, with subsequent permanent damage to sensory cells and neurons resulting in irreversible cell death.[1] The effect of aminoglycosides may also be latent due to slower endolymphatic drug clearance when compared with the serum. Patients who have undergone systemic therapy with aminoglycosides should be monitored for ototoxicity for up to 6 months after treatment.

It is important to take a family history of ototoxicity in patients where aminoglycoside treatment is planned. Some patients are genetically prone to aminoglycoside ototoxocity due to a mutation (A1555G) in the mitochondrial 12S ribosomal RNA gene, which causes a defect in mitochondrial protein synthesis.[2]

Many topical antibiotic drops used commonly in the ear contain aminoglycosides, as they are effective against common ear pathogens such as *Pseudomonas aeruginosa*. They can be safely used in the ear with an intact tympanic membrane (TM) without any risk of ototoxicity. Where the middle ear is open due to a perforation of the TM or the presence of a ventilation tube, there is the potential for ototoxicity due to drug permeability through the round window. However, their use in this situation is still justified as ototoxicity is infrequent (incidence ≤1:10,000), particularly in the presence of infection where inflamed, oedematous mucosa may act as a barrier to transportation across the round window. The justification for using topical aminoglycosides over other preparations (such as fluoroquinolones, which are not ototoxic) should be explained to the patient and a baseline audiogram should be performed if possible.[3]

LOOP DIURETICS

The most commonly used drugs in this group include furosemide, ethacrynic acid and bumetadine. These drugs may have an effect on the striae vascularis of the cochlea, causing an ionic gradient shift between the endolymph of the scala media and the perilymph of the scala tympani and scala vestibuli. The result is epithelial oedema of the striae vascularis. The incidence of ototoxicity in patients taking loop diuretics is 6–7%, with tinnitus and disequilibrium being the main symptoms experienced. The effect is dose-dependent and usually reversible, but may be irreversible in patients with renal failure or in those receiving very high doses.

PLATINUM-BASED CHEMOTHERAPEUTICS

Cisplatin and, to a lesser degree, carboplatin cause ototoxicity through free radical generation in the striae vascularis, resulting in death of OHCs, especially in the basal turn of the cochlea.

Patients may complain of tinnitus and hearing loss, which is usually bilateral, progressive and permanent. Ototoxicity can occur several days to months after administration, especially with cisplatin, which permanently binds to plasma proteins and can be detected in the blood for up to 6 months. Conversely, carboplatin does not bind to protein and is more readily cleared by the kidneys.

Patients receiving these drugs should have a baseline audiogram before starting each cycle and then periodically throughout their treatment. Therapy in subsequent cycles can then be titrated according to any ototoxicity experienced previously.[4] Patients should continue to have audiograms for at least 6 months following therapy due to the possibility of latent symptom onset. Noise exposure should also be avoided for at least 6 months.

SALICYLATES

The incidence of ototoxicity with salicylate use is approximately 1%. Salicylates such as aspirin rapidly enter the endolymph and may cause temporary SNHL and tinnitus through an effect on the spiral ganglion neurons of the cochlea as opposed to a direct effect on the OHCs.[5] Effects are likely to be multifactorial and do not result in morphological changes to the cochlea. Hearing loss and tinnitus progressively worsen with increasing aspirin dosage and with increasing concentrations of total and unbound plasma salicylate concentrations. The therapeutic range over which these symptoms occur is 30–300 mg/l, equivalent to single doses of 300–1,000 mg of aspirin. When used for its anti-platelet effects, plasma concentrations rarely rise above 10 mg/l and the degree of ototoxicity caused at this level is thought to be very low.[6]

QUININE

This antimalarial, which is also commonly used in the treatment of restless leg syndrome, can cause tinnitus, vertigo and reversible SNHL. This may occur at effective doses within therapeutic range, usually at the maximal plasma quinine concentration.[7] It is thought to cause vasoconstriction and a decrease in cochlear blood flow and reversible alterations of the OHCs. SNHL is typically high frequency and often not noticed by the patient.

CONCLUSION

Ototoxicity is a side-effect of many commonly used medications and its incidence is often underestimated. Ototoxicity is largely dependent on drug dose and renal function and ototoxic drugs should be used with care in the elderly. In instances where the indications for drug usage outweigh the risk of ototoxicity, appropriate counselling and audiometric monitoring should be offered, especially where the ototoxicity is likely to be permanent.

REFERENCES

1 Selimoglu E (2007) Aminoglycoside-induced ototoxicity. *Curr Pharm Des* **13**:119–126.
2 Casano RA, Johnson DF, Bykhovskaya Y *et al.* (1999) Inherited susceptibility to aminoglycoside ototoxicity: genetic heterogeneity and clinical implications. *Am J Otolaryngol* **20**:151–156.

3 Phillips JS, Yung MW, Burton MJ *et al.* (2007) Evidence review and ENT-UK consensus report for the use of aminoglycoside-containing ear drops in the presence of an open middle ear. *Clin Otolaryngol* **32:**330–336.

4 Fausti SA, Henry JA, Schaffer HI *et al.* (1993) High-frequency monitoring for early detection of cisplatin ototoxicity. *Arch Otolaryngol Head Neck Surg* **119:**661–666.

5 Wei L, Ding D, Salvi R (2010) Salicylate-induced degeneration of cochlea spiral ganglion neurons-apoptosis signaling. *Neuroscience* **168:**288–299.

6 Day RO, Graham GG, Bieri D *et al.* (1989) Concentration-response relationships for salicylate-induced ototoxicity in normal volunteers. *Br J Clin Pharmacol* **28:**695–702.

7 Jung TT, Rhee CK, Lee CS, Park YS, Choi DC. Ototoxicity of salicylate, nonsteroidal antiinflammatory drugs, and quinine. *Otolaryngol Clin North Am.* 1993;**26:**791–810.

23

AUDITORY BRAINSTEM IMPLANTS

Simon R.M. Freeman

Contents

INTRODUCTION

The auditory brainstem implant (ABI) is a device that provides hearing sensation to bilaterally, profoundly deafened patients when a cochlear implant is unsuitable. This is due to damaged or non-functional cochlear nerves or non-implantable cochleas. It is identical to a cochlear implant except that the stimulating electrode array is paddle-shaped and is placed directly on the cochlear nucleus, which lies in the floor of the foramen of Luschka in the lateral recess of the fourth ventricle of the brainstem (**Figure 23.1**).

INDICATIONS

The main indication is for post-lingually deafened patients with neurofibromatosis type 2 (NF2), an autosomal dominant genetic condition with an incidence of 1 in 33,000, which leads to bilateral vestibular schwannomas and subsequent destruction of the cochlear nerves.[1,2] Other indications include severe cochlear obliteration from otosclerosis or meningitis preventing effective cochlear implantation, head injury with bilateral cochlear nerve avulsion or in pre-lingually deafened young children with cochlear nerve deficiency or extreme degrees of inner ear dysplasia.[3,4]

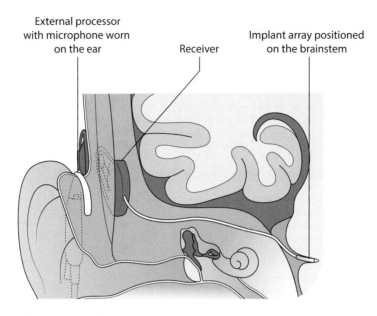

External processor with microphone worn on the ear

Receiver

Implant array positioned on the brainstem

Figure 23.1. Auditory brainstem implant.

SURGERY

Placement of the device is carried out through either a translabyrinthine or retrosigmoid route to the cerebellopontine angle. In young children, the latter approach is favoured as it reduces the risk of late device infection secondary to otitis media and surgical complications due to congenital abnormalities of the temporal bone. Placement can be carried out at the time of tumour removal in NF2 patients.

The major complication rate is estimated at approximately 1% and includes the risk of cranial nerve damage (facial, glossopharyngeal or vagal), cerebrospinal fluid leak, meningitis, intracranial bleeding, stroke and even risk to life.[5]

PROGRAMMING AND NON-AUDITORY STIMULATION

A cochlear implant works so well because the cochlea is tonotopic (high frequencies stimulate the basal turn and low frequencies stimulate the apical turn), meaning that replicating speech patterns is relatively straightforward. Unfortunately, the anatomical position of the cochlear nucleus and its tonotopicity is much less predictable, so accurate speech programming is more difficult. Adults who have learned speech prior to becoming deaf can give feedback to provide an idea of the pitch given by

different electrodes, although they usually find this very difficult. For children who have never heard sounds and have no concept of pitch perception, it is even more difficult to reproduce speech patterns.

An additional problem is that of non-auditory stimulation, where neighbouring cranial nerves are inadvertently stimulated by the implant. This can produce uncomfortable sensations such as dizziness, muscle twitching in the face, throat or tongue or discomfort anywhere in the body including the distal limbs; some electrodes on the device will inevitably need to be turned off. While adults may be able to communicate the fact that they are getting non-auditory stimulation, young children may not, necessitating even greater care during programming.

OUTCOME

Outcomes with the ABI are notoriously variable.[1,2] Approximately 20–30% of adults will become non-users because so little benefit is gained or they cannot become accustomed to the auditory stimulation. Most will benefit from the ability to discriminate between environmental sounds, and a significant improvement in communication when using lip reading in combination with the ABI. Only about 10–20% are able to understand speech with the ABI alone.

In pre-lingually deaf children the ABI has only been in use for about 10 years, so evidence on outcomes is only starting to emerge.[3,4] Current advice is that the majority will continue to use sign language as their main form of communication but may be able to recognise some environmental and speech sounds. The ability to learn to speak would be limited, with poor speech intelligibility. A small proportion will get no benefit. There are reports of children around the world who are able to communicate with their ABI alone and have developed good speech. At the present time it is difficult to predict what the chance of this happening is, but it is likely to be rare. Results also suggest that where children have other developmental problems, then the benefit from the ABI is limited to environmental awareness only without recognition of different sounds.

REFERENCES

1 Matthies C, Brill S, Kaga K *et al.* (2013) Auditory brainstem implantation improves speech recognition in neurofibromatosis type II patients. *ORL J Otorhinolaryngol Relat Spec* **75(5):**282–295.

2 Schwartz MS, Otto SR, Shannon RV *et al.* (2008) Auditory brainstem implants. *Neurotherapeutics* **5(1):**128–136.

3 Freeman SR, Stivaros SM, Ramsden RT *et al.* (2013) The management of cochlear nerve deficiency. *Cochlear Implants Int* **14(Suppl 4):** S27–31.

4 Sennaroglu L, Colletti V, Manrique M *et al.* (2011) Auditory brainstem implantation in children and non-neurofibromatosis type 2 patients: a consensus statement. *Otol Neurotol* **32(2):**187–191.

5 Colletti V, Shannon RV, Carner M *et al.* (2010) Complications in auditory brainstem implant surgery in adults and children. *Otol Neurotol* **31(4):**558–564.

24 HEARING AIDS

Sarah Yorke-Smith & Elizabeth Hough

Contents

INTRODUCTION

Hearing aids (HAs) are a key part of audiological rehabilitation, and provide amplification of sound that can be tuned to an individual's hearing loss to increase audibility.

CANDIDACY FOR HEARING AIDS

Anyone with a hearing loss might be considered a candidate for HAs, since HAs have the potential to offer benefit by providing access to environmental and speech sounds that would otherwise be missed. For mild hearing losses, there may be insufficient listening benefit to make HAs worth wearing for many individuals. One exception is the use of HAs for sound enrichment for tinnitus, where people with very mild hearing losses can benefit (see Chapters 26 and 27: Hearing habilitation and rehabilitation in children and adults, respectively). For the most severe hearing losses, especially for speech distortion problems, it may be that HAs are not enough and implanted devices such as a cochlear implant should be considered. However, there is more to candidacy that hearing thresholds (**Figure 24.1**).

While HA technology is continually improving, HAs cannot fully compensate for hearing loss. Sensorineural hearing loss (SNHL) is most commonly associated with cochlear damage. This may lead not only to some sounds seeming quiet, but also to problems distinguishing various types of sounds. For example, cochlear damage may cause difficulties perceiving different sound frequencies and timings, and in some cases there may be 'dead' regions in the cochlea. Sound processed by a HA is delivered to the damaged cochlea, resulting in a poor representation of sound, mainly attributable to the cochlear impairment, but there may also be a reduction of fidelity associated with HA sound processing and reproduction. These effects may be experienced as difficulties recognising speech and problems hearing with background noise or in complex listening environments. Indeed, HAs tend to be least successful in cases where there is significant distortion in the hearing system (e.g. from cochlear or neural damage) or where significant auditory deprivation leads to a reduced ability to process sounds. Assisting the detection of speech in background noise remains a significant challenge in HA research. Given these limitations, and the importance of communication, HAs are generally set up to maximise speech recognition, and are often limited in how well they can process other types of sounds such as music.

Conductive hearing losses can be managed using HAs where not contraindicated (e.g. discharging ears). In this case, the device simply provides more volume to overcome the conductive component, but this can be limited due to feedback and reaching the maximum power output of the device. Alternative approaches might be surgical correction, bone-anchored hearing aids (BAHAs) or other implantable devices.

For bilateral hearing loss it is usual to prescribe HAs binaurally, although this depends on the individual's preference, listening needs, management of aids and any contraindications (**Figure 24.1**). Dynamic listening environments with competing sounds from different directions may favour binaural fitting more strongly than a relatively quiet world where the wearer has more chance to turn their aided ear towards the sound source.

For asymmetric hearing loss, the primary management might be to fit a HA in the poorer ear. However, this does not always lead to an improvement in communication if that ear has poor speech discrimination and aiding the better hearing ear or binaurally may be preferable. Where one ear has unaidable hearing due to severity of loss or poor speech discrimination, a CROS (contralateral routing of signal) aid can be used to route sound detected at the poor hearing ear to the better hearing ear, either via a wire or wirelessly (**Figure 24.2**). Alternatively, a BAHA can be used to pick up sound at the poor ear and deliver the sound by bone conduction to the better hearing cochlea.

It is good practice to reassesses HA candidacy over time as changes in hearing or general health may require revised HA settings or an overall change of plan.

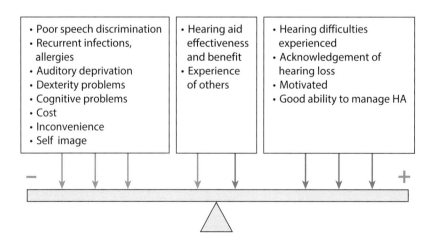

Figure 24.1. Factors affecting hearing aid candidacy and likely outcome. Negative factors on the left and positive factors on the right.

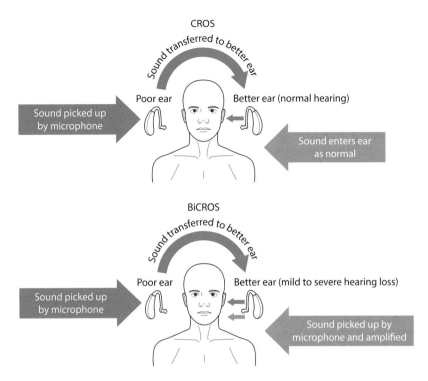

Figure 24.2. Illustrations of a CROS and a BiCROS hearing aid. A microphone placed behind or in the poorer ear picks up the surrounding sounds, then a transmitter sends the sounds (either via a wire or wirelessly) to the better hearing ear. The sounds are delivered to the better hearing ear directly (for a CROS aid) or amplified by a hearing aid (for a BiCROS aid), as appropriate to the hearing level of the better hearing ear.

HOW HEARING AIDS WORK

HAs may be selected from a range of styles and types (**Figures 24.3A–F**) on the basis of power, technical features, comfort, cost and appearance/cosmetic appeal. HAs are composed of the following parts (**Figure 24.4**):

- A microphone picks up sound and converts it to electrical signals.
- An amplifier and digital sound processor amplifies and processes the electrical signal.
- A receiver converts the amplified signal back to sound to be delivered to the ear.
- A battery powers the device.

SNHL is associated with loss of ability to hear quiet sounds, while loud sounds are perceived at about the same loudness as someone with normal hearing.

This leads to a reduced dynamic listening range and abnormal loudness growth (known as 'recruitment'). It is a challenge to fit HAs to give access to soft sounds without loud sounds becoming uncomfortable, but is usually achieved using 'wide dynamic range compression'. Rather than all sounds being amplified by the same amount (linear amplification used in older analogue HAs), less amplification is prescribed for sounds above an assigned point ('kneepoint') leading to a more normal growth of loudness and more comfortable listening (**Figure 24.5**). Maximum outputs of HAs are limited for safety and comfort.

The HA is programmed by the audiologist to fit a particular hearing loss according to a frequency-dependent prescription using information from

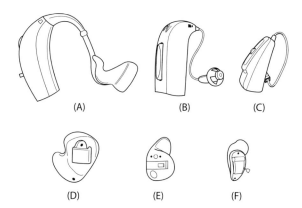

(A) (B) (C)

(D) (E) (F)

Figures 24.3A–F. Hearing aid styles. (A) Behind the ear. (B) Open fit behind the ear. (C) Receiver in the canal. (D) In the ear. (E) In the canal. (F) Completely in the canal. In addition, body worn hearing aids have an ear piece connected to a separate processor (not shown).

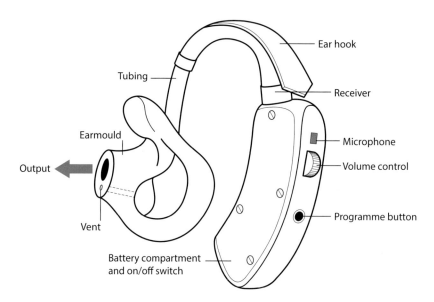

Figure 24.4. Diagram of a behind the ear hearing aid showing the components.

the audiogram. The sound profile can be verified and refined by performing real ear measurements (REMs), involving measuring HA performance inside the wearer's ear using a microphone attached to a thin pre-calibrated measurement tube inserted in the ear. REMs effectively take into account the individual's ear canal acoustic environment so that amplification can be modified as appropriate. Alternative predictive methods of estimating ear

canal acoustics can be used if REMs are not feasible (e.g. due to infection/occluding wax). Subjective checks of comfort and the individual's response to amplification complement the technical measurements. Speech mapping tools may also be employed to show how the HA amplifies speech sounds, so that the HA can be adjusted to optimise the audibility of speech sounds while evading loudness discomfort.

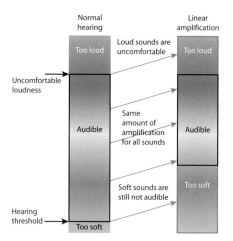
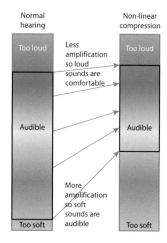

Figure 24.5. Compression. Reduced dynamic hearing range for hearing loss is shown. With linear amplification soft sounds are inaudible and loud sounds are uncomfortably loud. Non-linear compression can be applied so amplified sounds are audible and more comfortable.

Many types of HA (**Figures 24.3A, D–F**) are designed to fit the shape of the wearer's ear by taking an impression (or cast) of the ear using putty. The custom-fit HA or connecting earmoulds can be vented to modify acoustics, increase comfort, reduce infection risk (e.g. for perforated eardrums), improve perceived sound quality and reduce the sensation of 'occlusion' where the wearer's voice may sound 'boomy' or 'hollow'. Behind the ear HAs (**Figure 24.3A**) deliver sound through custom earmoulds connected to the HA via tubing (**Figure 24.4**). Earmould materials range from hard arcylics to soft silicones, and are selected to suit individuals based on hearing level, dexterity and likelihood of ear infections. Special coatings can be used where there is risk of allergy. Tightly fitting soft moulds may be needed for severe losses to minimise acoustic feedback. Open fit and receiver in the canal HAs (**Figures 24.3B, C**) do not require custom earmoulds and may be preferred for cosmetic reasons due to the narrow tubing or wire and discreet ear tip. They are particularly appropriate for mild to moderate high frequency losses with good low frequency hearing (often associated with presbycusis or noise-induced hearing loss) but can be challenging to fit for more severe or less common hearing loss configurations. 'In the ear' style HAs (**Figures 24.3D–F**) can fit a range of hearing losses, but the smallest devices may be limited in power, features and size of controls and are subject to the shape and size of the individual's ear.

Examples of HA features include:

- Different programmes (e.g. telecoil).
- Volume control.
- Feedback management: electronic mechanisms designed to reduce the problem of feedback (whistling caused by some of the HA output getting back to the microphone and being re-amplified).
- Directional microphones: attenuate sounds from some directions (e.g. sound [speech] is picked up from the front and sound [noise] from behind is partially suppressed).
- Adaptive listening: automatic directional microphones/programmes (may improve hearing and comfort for speech in noise situations).
- Frequency compression: high frequency sounds are compressed into a lower frequency region thus increasing access to high frequency speech cues.

Table 24.1 includes a list of common problems with HAs (both behind the ear and in front of the ear), and possible causes and solutions for trouble shooting purposes.

Table 24.1. Hearing aid problems with possible causes and solutions.

Common HA problems	Possible cause	Solutions
No sound or reduced sound	Dead battery	Replace battery
	Blocked sound outlet	Clean
	HA fault	Return to HA provider for repair/replacement
Reduced sound or poor sound quality	Blocked HA filters	Replace filters or return to HA provider
	Moisture in HA	Use drying kit or leave in a warm place to dry
	Behind the ear HA tubing blocked, damaged, stiff or condensation in tubing	Clean or replace tubing
Acoustic feedback ('whistling')	Wax build up in the ear canal	Arrange wax removal
	Loose or incorrectly inserted earmould/HA	Reinsert HA or return to HA provider for new earmould/HA
	Volume too high	Reduce volume or return to HA provider
Battery runs out quickly	Using wireless connectivity frequently	Normal behaviour
	HA feedback manager working too hard	See acoustic feedback above
	Faulty battery or HA	Replace battery or return to HA provider
Sounds 'tinny'	Not used to hearing high frequencies	Advice on acclimatisation or fine-tune HA by HA provider
Sounds 'boomy'	Not used to hearing low frequencies or occlusion effect from ears being blocked	Advice on acclimatisation or fine-tune HA by HA provider
HA uncomfortable in ear	Incorrectly inserted, poor fit	Reinsert or return to HA provider
	Irritation or infection	Seek medical assistance

FURTHER READING

Dillon H (2012) *Hearing Aids*, 2nd edn. Boomerang Press, Sydney.

Gelfand SA (2001) *Essentials of Audiology*, 2nd edn. Thieme, New York.

Moore, BCJ (2007) *Cochlear Hearing Loss*, 2nd edn. John Wiley and Sons, Chichester.

25 HEARING THERAPY

Elizabeth Hough & Sarah Yorke-Smith

Contents

INTRODUCTION

Hearing therapy is part of hearing rehabilitation aimed at helping people and their families come to terms with their hearing loss and effectively manage their listening difficulties. This can include lay personnel adjustment counselling (listening to the emotional content and providing support)[1], informational counselling (understanding how hearing works and the implications of hearing loss) and working together to develop positive strategies and skills.

HEARING LOSS AND PSYCHOSOCIAL ISSUES

Hearing loss does not only lead to practical difficulties but there is also a strong emotional dimension. Hearing can be considered on three basic levels[2]:

1 Primitive level. Hearing background sounds such as a ticking clock, traffic or the sounds of other people in the background. This gives us the feeling of being part of a living world and the absence of this level of hearing can lead to depression.

2 Warning level. Hearing sounds that convey information such as an alarm, doorbell or localisation of sounds. This gives us a sense of security and the absence can lead to feelings of anxiety and insecurity.

3 Symbolic level. Hearing sounds for language and communication. Without effective communication a range of difficulties may arise:

● Frustration and tension in the home.
● Difficulties at work, which may limit career progression.
● Difficulties using the phone effectively, which impede conducting business or limit opportunities for social contact.
● Difficulty listening in background noise and groups leading to misunderstandings, embarrassment and avoiding contact, leading to isolation and loneliness.

Loss of hearing can also be considered as having a concomitant grieving process. Understanding the grieving process and the individual's emotional response, which can depend on changing circumstances throughout life, helps clinicians provide an appropriate response to an individual with hearing loss.

Hearing therapy can help a person understand how their hearing difficulties are affected by internal and external factors and help develop positive coping strategies (**Figure 25.1**). The Table below shows examples of when hearing therapy is appropriate and when referral to other services is required.

Hearing therapy appropriate	Referral to other services required
Difficulties accepting hearing loss or change in hearing. Negative attitudes towards hearing loss or hearing aids	Psychological conditions associated with hearing loss (e.g. anxiety, depression, post-traumatic stress disorder)
Participation limitation caused by hearing loss. Lack of confidence or motivation	Psychological problems not related to hearing loss
Coping with increased listening effort. Maladaptive coping strategies	Tinnitus and hyperacusis management. Multidisciplinary specialist service (medical, audiological and psychological) is recommended
Listening difficulties in the absence of hearing loss (or for minimal hearing loss)	Non-organic hearing loss. Where psychological management is required, this should be referred to a qualified psychologist
Understanding and accepting limitations of living with a hearing loss	Auditory processing disorder diagnosis and management

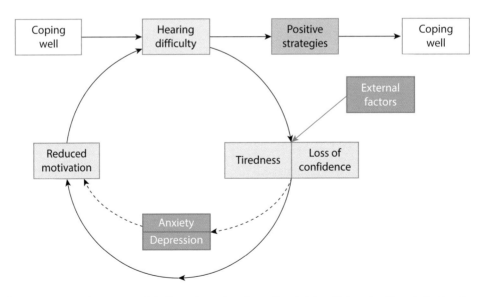

Figure 25.1. Hearing therapy model. (Based on data from Cambridge University Hospitals Hearing Therapy Team.)

HEARING THERAPY MANAGEMENT

The structure of a management plan is tailored to the individual and their needs within the framework of local service provision. Basic audiological counselling, communication training and problem solving should be performed routinely as part of the adult rehabilitation (hearing aid) pathway, but more complex cases should be referred to a specialist audiologist or therapist. A therapist can also deliver communication training to individuals, families or in a group setting. Auditory training consists of exercises aimed at improving listening skills and can be delivered by therapists or, more commonly, as computer-based training. Training programmes are available to help develop listening and communication skills for people with different severities of hearing loss including people with normal hearing who experience listening difficulties in noise.

Therapists also have a key role in signposting or referring to other services. The session number and duration can vary, with a single hour session and follow-up a few months later being appropriate for many patients through to intensive auditory rehabilitation programmes for new cochlear implant users.

REFERENCES

1 Clark JG, Martin FN (1994) *Effective Counseling in Audiology: Perspectives and Practice*. Prentice-Hall, New Jersey.
2 Ramsdell DA (1978) The psychology of the hard of hearing and deafened adult. In: *Hearing and Deafness*. (eds. H Davis, SR Silverman) Holt, Rinehart & Winston, New York.

26 HEARING HABILITATION IN CHILDREN

Victoria H. Parfect & Sarah Yorke-Smith

Developments in newborn hearing screening and diagnostic auditory brainstem response assessments have meant that hearing impairment can be identified within weeks of birth. Aural impressions taken at the point of diagnosis allow hearing aids to be fitted within weeks of confirmation of a hearing loss. The aim of early habilitation is to normalise communication and social development by facilitating auditory system development. Effective early amplification promotes development of the auditory pathway by enriching auditory exposure and strengthening neural plasticity. Paediatric habilitation continues throughout childhood with the support emphasis shifting from parent to child to adolescent before transition to adult services.

Once a child is diagnosed with a hearing loss, referrals are made in agreement with families to audiology, hearing support services, ENT, paediatricians and for aetiological investigations (e.g. ophthalmology, genetics) to inform habilitation planning, hearing aid selection and family counselling. Families are also signposted to charity organisations for support and information.

Regular paediatric audiology reviews ensure appropriate hearing aid prescription via:

- Detailed history focused on hearing aid use, including difficulties or faults with amplification, common home/education auditory environments and symptoms including otorrhoea, otalgia, balance, tinnitus and allergies to materials.
- Regular aural impressions (can be weekly for infants).
- Hearing assessments to define ear and frequency specific hearing thresholds, the configuration and nature of loss.
- Verification of hearing aid fitting using real ear measurements to account for individual ear canal acoustic changes.
- Validation using questionnaires to assess functional outcomes in the home and educational environments.
- Functional speech assessments using phonemes, single words or sentences tests utilising toys and pictures to assess detection and discrimination of speech in quiet and noise and for unaided/aided conditions.

Additionally, hearing aids are adjusted regularly throughout childhood in response to:

- Growth, causing acoustic changes of the ear canal and/or the earmould venting options.
- Environmental demands requiring different programmes or features, for example FM and/or loop system compatibility.
- Requirements for assistive listening devices giving access to technology, music or for safety.
- Routine upgrades with advances in hearing aid technology.

It is important that parents are taught hearing aid maintenance and methods of assessing aided hearing function in their children, to quickly identify faults in the technology or changes in hearing.

In the UK, hearing support teachers are a critical bridge between children, families, schools and audiologists to facilitate hearing aid use, education and effective amplification.

Early amplification, support and monitoring are key to achieving the goals of paediatric hearing habilitation. Family engagement is critical. The diagnosis of a hearing loss can be devastating. At diagnosis, we ask parents to understand the complex anatomy and neurophysiology of the hearing system, while addressing the emotional impact of the diagnosis. While our goal is to provide effective amplification and constantly review this in response to family observations, investigations, assessments and changing technology, it is the family that manages hearing impairment on a daily basis. It is therefore essential that alongside the technology, we give families the information and skills to have confidence to take an active part in this process to enable them to support their child and drive effective early amplification.

27 HEARING REHABILITATION IN ADULTS

Sarah Yorke-Smith & Elizabeth Hough

Contents

INTRODUCTION

Rehabilitation for deafness goes far beyond addressing the physical impairment. Effective rehabilitation does not just involve a hearing aid (HA) fitting, but also helping the individual understand their hearing loss. Rehabilitation enables them to become effective and confident HA users, makes them aware of beneficial services and equipment as well as developing the skills to make the most of their hearing in a range of everyday situations.

USING HEARING AIDS

After a HA has been provided a process of 'acclimatization' is required for the wearer to adapt to a new way of listening, and this process may be hindered in cases of auditory deprivation or where there is low personal motivation to persevere with wearing the HA continuously. Hearing therapy (see Chapter 25: Hearing therapy) may be needed to help an individual to come to terms with their hearing loss and persevere with wearing HAs both in private and public settings, and hence assist the wearer with maintaining a healthy level of activity and participation to avoid social isolation. Common problems with HAs include issues with physical comfort, cosmesis and sound and noise discomfort. Ongoing care, including counselling, technical assistance and regular maintenance (e.g. replacement of earmould tubing to avoid wax/moisture blockages), may be required to optimise hearing and effective HA use.

Sensitive comprehensive care may be required where additional factors such as cognitive impairment, dementia, vision or dexterity issues are involved. In these cases, it is key to provide information and services in an accessible way and involve family or carers where appropriate.

HEARING AID BENEFITS AND LIMITATIONS

Hearing aid benefits (outcome) can be measured using questionnaires. A number of questionnaires are available such as COSI (Client Oriented Scale of Improvement), which can be useful to gauge individual benefit and assist with counselling and the design of rehabilitation approaches. Tests measuring hearing levels and speech intelligibility can be performed in an aided or unaided state, and with or without background noise to manage expectations, to further assess HA benefit and guide treatment.

Hearing loss often leads to difficulties listening in background noise since it is not only associated with a reduction in volume, but also reduced ability to pick out the wanted sound (signal) and ignore unwanted sounds (noise). This difficulty is not fully ameliorated by HAs and successful rehabilitation should help optimise communication.

Hearing loss can lead to deficits in sound localisation, particularly in cases of significant asymmetrical hearing, since most of the ability to localise sounds is attributable to two ears working together, and this issue is currently not resolved by HAs. In these cases, rehabilitation should include counselling warning of potential difficulties with localisation and discussing possible safety measures such as maximising use of available vision to locate sounds such as traffic.

COMMUNICATION STRATEGIES

Discussing personalised communication tactics is recommended in cases of hearing loss, regardless of whether a HA has been fitted, since this may help to reduce activity limitations and participation restrictions by improving signal to noise ratios and helping an individual to feel more confident in difficult listening situations. Tactics may include manipulating the environment to reduce background noise, limit reverberation (e.g. by soft furnishings) and keeping the speaker and listener close and facing each other in a well-lit environment (to facilitate lip reading). It is preferable for the speaker to speak slowly, clearly and provide the context from the beginning and avoid covering their mouth, and for the listener to assertively explain how the speaker can help and to know conversation repair strategies (**Figure 27.1**). Family-centered care is appropriate when addressing communication tactics, since communication is a two-way process and will require the speaker and listener to work together.

HEARING AIDS AND TINNITUS

Fitting HAs is often beneficial for people with troublesome tinnitus, even when hearing loss is minimal. Helping an individual to engage with a rich external sound environment may assist shifting the focus away from internal sounds. An alternative to a conventional HA is a 'tinnitus combination device', which combines amplification with sound therapy (sound generator). Sound therapy, counselling and relaxation can also form part of a rehabilitation programme for tinnitus (see Chapter 29: Tinnitus).

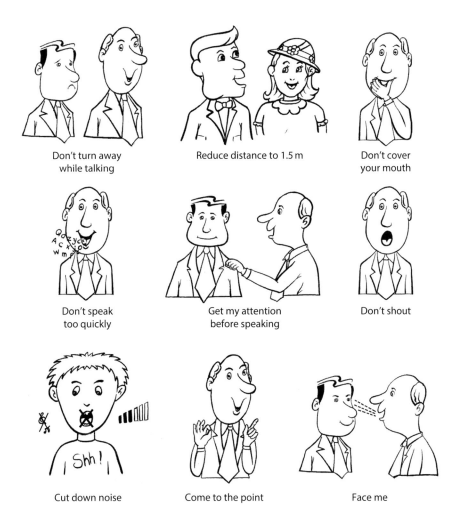

Don't turn away while talking

Reduce distance to 1.5 m

Don't cover your mouth

Don't speak too quickly

Get my attention before speaking

Don't shout

Cut down noise

Come to the point

Face me

Figure 27.1. Communication tactics.

FURTHER READING

Dillon H (2012) *Hearing Aids*, 2nd edn. Boomerang Press, Sydney.

Schow RL, Nerbonne MA (2013) *Introduction to Audiologic Rehabilitation*, 6th edn. Pearson, Boston.

28 ADDITIONAL SUPPORT FOR PATIENTS WITH HEARING LOSS

Elizabeth Hough & Sarah Yorke-Smith

Contents

INTRODUCTION

While hearing aids (HAs) can be of great benefit, there remain some challenges of living with a hearing loss that cannot be met by HAs alone. Provision of these services may exist through social care initiatives, schemes for people with disabilities to access employment or through groups such as veterans.

ASSISTIVE LISTENING DEVICES

Alerting equipment is available for the following warning sounds:

- Phone ringing.
- Doorbell.
- Alarm clock.
- Fire/smoke alarm.
- Baby alarm.

Alerts can be made more noticeable by:

- Louder, longer or lower pitched alarm.
- Flashing light.
- Vibrating pager.
- Portable devices.

- Vibrating pads that fit under the pillow for alerting at night.

Using the telephone can be a particular problem at home, work and for mobile phones due to the reduced sound quality and loss of visual cues. Helpful phone features include:

- Amplification.
- Tone control.
- Speakerphone.
- Telecoil compatibility.
- Clear sound reproduction.
- Wireless connectivity to hearing aids.

For people unable to use a conventional phone alternatives include:

- SMS text.
- Text phones.
- Text relay or captioning service.
- Video communication.
- Email/fax/letter/face-to-face communication.

Personal listeners help the user focus on the person talking (**Figure 28.1**). A transmitter equipped with a microphone is placed near the sound source, which wirelessly sends information to a receiver worn by the HA user. FM systems (radio aids) use ear level radio receivers plugged directly into the HAs and are widely used in an educational setting.

High-volume television/music can cause difficulties in the family and with neighbours. The following may help:

- Loop systems (also known as induction loops, telecoil or T systems).
- Television listener.
- Wireless streamer or personal listener.
- Subtitles (may also be available at cinema/theatre).

A loop system works by picking up the sound source from a microphone or input from audio equipment (e.g. television, personal music player). The signal is sent to an amplifier, which is connected to a loop of wire usually around the room perimeter. This wire loop generates a magnetic field, which can be picked up by a small loop of wire in HAs equipped with a telecoil programme (**Figure 28.2**). This system may be installed in home, work or educational environments as well as in other public buildings (e.g. cinema, theatres, places of worship and shop counters indicated with a sign) (**Figure 28.2**). HAs are increasingly able to connect to wireless (Bluetooth) equipment either directly or via an intermediate device called a streamer.

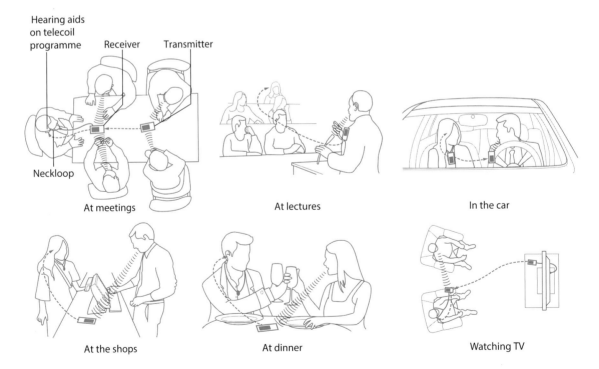

Figure 28.1. Examples of personal listener usage.

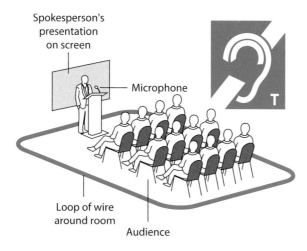

Figure 28.2. Example loop system and loop sign.

Hearing Dogs are an alternative to equipment. They are trained to alert their owners to a range of environmental warning and alerting sounds and may also provide companionship and give people confidence to enter unfamiliar situations.

ADDITIONAL SUPPORT SERVICES

Rehabilitation programmes and groups can help people and their families adjust to living with a significant hearing loss by providing:

- Information about services and equipment.
- Strategies for dealing with communication problems.
- Shared experiences with peers.
- Meetings role models.
- Lip-reading training.
- Communication strategies.
- HA care and maintenance.
- Talks and social activities with communication support.
- Tinnitus support groups.

Local, national and international voluntary organisations also have an important role including:

- Information and advice.
- Campaigning for better services and access.
- Raising awareness.
- Fundraising.
- Supporting research.

Communication support services are mainly used in work or educational institutions but can also increase accessibility of seminars or entertainment. Support may be in the form of:

- Note takers.
- Speech to text live captioning.
- Sign language interpretation.
- Foreign language interpretation (communication barriers can increase when non-native languages are involved).

One-to-one support can be helpful for people with hearing loss facing additional problems for example:

- Advocacy and help managing everyday life.
- Mental health support (increased risk for people with significant hearing loss).

Deaf associations are traditionally run by and for culturally deaf sign language users (e.g. British sign Language [BSL] or American Sign Language [ASL]), but some also provide services for people with a hearing loss who communicate aurally. The focus tends to be on social, entertainment and educational activities.

Deaf sign language users may use HAs and equipment to access warning sounds. Although some are accomplished lip-readers, auditory communication and voice may be rarely used. In some cases, written language skills may be limited as English would be a second language. Where these individuals interact with the auditory world, sign language interpreters are required. On-line interpreting can be useful for unanticipated interactions.

FURTHER READING

Derebery MJ, Luxford WM (2010) *Hearing Loss: The Otolaryngologist's Guide to Amplification*. Plural Publishing, San Diego.

Schow, RL, Nerbonne MA (2013) *Introduction to Audiologic Rehabilitation*, 6th edn. Pearson, Boston.

29 TINNITUS

David M. Baguley

Contents

INTRODUCTION

The management of a patient with troublesome tinnitus can be a challenge for even an experienced clinician. This chapter aims to describe the fundamentals of diagnosis and treatment, and to briefly reflect on future hopes.

The word tinnitus derives from the Latin *tinnire* (to ring), and is colloquially known as ringing in the ears, although in fact patients use many words to describe the experience, commonly hissing, buzzing and grinding. For some there is a distinct pulsatile component to the sound. The tinnitus sound can be perceived in one ear, or both, or centrally in the head. Rarely, a patient may describe a point of origin external but close to their body.

Tinnitus is a symptom rather than a condition in itself, and the clinician should attempt to exclude any treatable pathology with audiological and radiological investigations. This should be undertaken without further alarming the patient – those with troublesome tinnitus are already anxious and distressed almost by definition.

An associated symptom is that of hyperacusis, or reduced sound tolerance. This is present in approximately 40% of patients with tinnitus (both adults and children), and is discussed in detail in Chapter 30 (Hyperacusis).

EPIDEMIOLOGY AND NATURAL HISTORY

There are many studies that report the prevalence of tinnitus, but unfortunately the quality of the literature is not high, and is marked by many different definitions concerning the severity and duration of tinnitus. In adults the most robust data indicate that about 30% of the UK population experience tinnitus at one time or another, 10% are bothered by it, and 2% are severely affected, experiencing insomnia, poor concentration and emotional distress. Incidence data is sparse, but indications are that between 2% and 4% of the UK adult population have sought specialist advice about tinnitus.

There are also indications that the experience of background noise in the ears and head of humans in silence is very common. This has led to a view that many experience tinnitus-like sensations, but do not find them bothersome, and that filtering mechanisms normal render us unaware of such sensations.

Less information is available for children, but it is reported that the incidence is similar to that for adults. Tinnitus is more common in children who have a hearing loss than those who do not (whether sensorineural or conductive) and more common still in those who acquire a hearing loss rather than being born with it. Far fewer children are seen clinically with tinnitus than adults, and it is not known whether this is due to a paucity of interested clinicians and service, lack of knowledge amongst GPs or perhaps children being less distressed by the symptom, although when a child is distressed this can be severe. Also of interest is the fact that few adults complaining of tinnitus report that it began in childhood.

The prevalence of tinnitus is more common in women than men, and rises with age, hearing loss, noise exposure and smoking. These are not independent factors, and there may be complex associations. It is also slightly but persistently more common in the left ear than the right. Many people with tinnitus experience more than one noise, and the perception may be complex. It is quite common for tinnitus to undergo somatic modulation, in that the intensity or pitch may change with head movement or teeth clenching.

Many people are curious rather than distressed about their tinnitus at onset, and the characteristic agitation and vigilance may develop over time. The current understanding is that all mammals have an auditory danger detection system, interweaving hearing with systems of reaction, emotion and learning, and that tinnitus activates these functions and then is perceived as intense and distressing. The vicious circles that can develop in a person with troublesome tinnitus are illustrated in **Figure 29.1**.

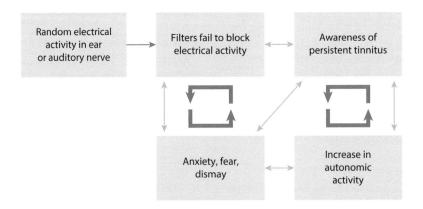

Figure 29.1. Vicious circles associated with tinnitus. (Adapted with permission from McKenna L, Baguley DM, McFerran D (2010) *Living with Tinnitus and Hyperacusis*. Sheldon Press, London.)

Table 29.1. Medical conditions associated with hearing loss, and key features.

Condition	Key features
Presbyacusis	Progressive, usually symmetrical age-related SNHL
Ototoxic hearing loss	Enquire regarding aminoglycoside antibiotics, non-steroidal anti-inflammatories, quinine, chemotherapy
Noise-induced hearing loss	Characteristic notch at 4–6 kHz
Idiopathic sudden SNHL	Treat as medical emergency with steroids within 14 days of onset. Salvage treatment with intratympanic steroids occasionally effective
Ménière's Disease	Low frequency fluctuating SNHL, episodic rotary vertigo. Tinnitus may be low frequency and fluctuant
Glomus tympanicum/jugulare	Pulse-synchronous tinnitus
Otosclerosis	Progressive conductive hearing loss in middle life. May be unilateral or bilateral
Vestibular schwannoma	Asymmetric hearing loss and unilateral tinnitus
Benign intracranial hypertension	Tinnitus may be pulsatile and worse on lying down
Middle ear myoclonus	Irregular fluttering sensation in ear, modulated by anxiety and/or stress. Usually unilateral

SNHL, sensorineural hearing loss.

Once it has become troublesome the natural history is influenced by the aetiology of the tinnitus. Common medical conditions associated with tinnitus are listed in **Table 29.1**. If associated with otological pathology, such as progressive otosclerosis, Ménière's disease or a growing vestibular schwannoma, the tinnitus progresses also and becomes more severe. If idiopathic or associated with a stable sensorineural hearing loss, the patient may habituate, becoming progressively less distressed and sometimes less aware of the tinnitus. The analogy is with a person who lives close by a railway line, but who has become unaware of the frequent train sounds. The phenomenon of habituation underpins current approaches to tinnitus therapy. As will be described, these vary in emphasis, but all aim to down rate the reaction to tinnitus, both behavioural and emotional, and to reduce the starkness of the tinnitus.

MECHANISMS

Patients will often ask "what actually is my tinnitus?". While the answer may vary with aetiology, there are a number of mechanisms current under research consideration. The first is an increase in the spontaneous activity within the auditory pathway, although in experimental studies, interventions that cause abrupt hearing loss decrease this activity in the cochlear nerve. The suggestion then is that this decrease disinhibits the central auditory system, so that spontaneous activity arises in higher nuclei. Another possibility is that spontaneous activity becomes self-correlated or synchronous, and thus perceived as signal rather than background noise. These proposed mechanisms can be summarised for patients as tinnitus being 'background noise in the hearing brain'.

INVESTIGATION AND DIAGNOSIS

Tinnitus should be considered as an indication of otological pathology until that has been excluded. A careful history is indicated, the essential elements of which are listed in **Table 29.2**.

Otoscopy and audiometry (air and bone) are essential. In cases of unilateral tinnitus and/or asymmetric hearing, MRI is mandatory unless contraindicated to exclude a vestibular schwannoma. Where there is a pulsatile component to the tinnitus, MRI can be augmented by a CT venogram of the head and neck to exclude vascular malformation and venous outflow obstruction suggestive of idiopathic intracranial hypertension.

Some patients complaining of tinnitus may also report a fluttering sensation in their ear, which may co-vary with anxiety or stress; in such cases middle ear myoclonus should be suspected, usually arising from the tensor tympani muscle.

Table 29.2. Essential elements of a tinnitus history.

Onset of tinnitus and context of illness or life events
Nature and site of tinnitus sounds
Patient perceived cause
Variability of tinnitus
Exacerbating factors (including stress, anxiety, noise)
Ameliorating factors
Impact on sleep
Prescribed medication
General medical history
Symptoms associated with tinnitus
Impact of tinnitus on daily life and mood state
Noise exposure (present and historical)
Hearing handicap
Reduced sound tolerance
General medical history

TREATMENT

While no effective treatment to abolish tinnitus yet exists, there are effective management techniques for which the evidence base is growing. Where there is a hearing loss, surgical correction if possible, and hearing aid amplification if not, is helpful. Some modern hearing aids have the option of sound generator use, either wide-band or environmental sound, and this can reduce the starkness of tinnitus. In a person with normal hearing, the sound generator option can be used to blend with the tinnitus, at a loudness described as the mixing point, rather than to mask the tinnitus as had previously been utilised, with little benefit.

Careful counselling about the cause of tinnitus and explaining the impact is indicated. When a person is agitated and stressed, relaxation therapy is used, and a specific technique called Progressive Muscle Relaxation can be used. The exercise involves systematic tensing and relaxing of muscle groups,

directed by a CD, and is particularly useful in patients who appreciate the need to relax but do not know where to start.

When insomnia is evident, the use of bedside environmental sound therapy is indicated, using a digital sound generator to play sounds such as gentle rainfall, the ocean, woods and birds either by the bedside or via a sound pillow with embedded loudspeakers. The aim is to blend the environmental sound with the tinnitus (rather than to mask it entirely), and most sleeping partners tolerate the technique well. In more severe instances of insomnia, sleep management techniques can be utilised, including the unspoken repetition of nonsense syllables, and sleep hygiene, which involves rising at the same time each morning, whatever the night may have held in terms of sleep. A small number of patients find that sleep medication is required, and a strategy of using the hypnotic properties of low-dose amitriptyline may be preferred to stronger dependence-inducing medications.

The vast majority of tinnitus clinicians use these techniques, with different emphases. The term Tinnitus Retraining Therapy is used for a protocol using sound generators and explanation, and Cognitive Behaviour Therapy, a form of psychotherapy, changes beliefs about the tinnitus, but also utilises sound therapy. Evidence indicates that good treatment outcomes and low relapse rates are achieved by combining sound and psychological strategies.[1]

Self-help has a major role, and can involve self-initiated treatments leading to relaxation (such as massage or acupuncture) or the use of structured self-help material.[2]

FUTURE TREATMENTS

The present situation regarding the treatment of tinnitus is not satisfactory for either patients or clinicians, and major efforts are underway internationally to develop effective interventions. These include drugs, with cochlear and brainstem target sites, transcranial magnetic cortical stimulation and new approaches to sound therapy. Additionally, the psychology community are investigating the clinical utility of mindfulness meditation and the 'third wave' approaches to Cognitive Behaviour Therapy, specifically Acceptance and Commitment Therapy. There are significant challenges in tinnitus research, including the heterogeneity of aetiology and reaction to tinnitus, and the need for robust and responsive outcome measures, but these are being addressed[3] and many in the field are cautiously optimistic.[4]

REFERENCES

1 Cima RF, Maes IH, Joore MA *et al.* (2012) Specialised treatment based on cognitive behaviour therapy versus usual care for tinnitus: a randomised controlled trial. *Lancet* **379(9830):**1951–1959.

2 McKenna L, Baguley DM, McFerran D (2010) *Living with Tinnitus and Hyperacusis.* Sheldon Press, London.

3 Landgrebe M, Azevedo A, Baguley D *et al.* (2012) Methodological aspects of clinical trials in tinnitus: a proposal for an international standard. *J Psychosom Res* **73(2):**112–121.

4 Baguley D, McFerran D, Hall D (2013) Tinnitus. *Lancet* **382(9904):**1600–1607.

30

HYPERACUSIS

Don J. McFerran

Contents

INTRODUCTION

We all experience sounds that we dislike. Sometimes this is because we perceive the sound as being too loud but at other times the problem may be the context, nature or character of the sound rather than its sound level. Chalk screeching down a blackboard, or the sound of vomiting are examples of sounds that most people find unpleasant, irrespective of the level. Tolerance to sound is not a fixed entity, varying not only with the nature of the sound but also with our mood and factors such as the amount of background noise. It is, therefore, difficult to define normal sound tolerance and by extension it is difficult to define what is abnormal. The study of impaired sound tolerance is an emergent field and there are many unanswered questions.

DEFINITIONS

▌ Hyperacusis

Hyperacusis is a word that can be used as an umbrella term to describe multiple types of impaired sound tolerance, but can also be used to denote a specific form of impaired sound tolerance. The following definitions have been used to describe this specific symptom:

- Unusual tolerance to ordinary environmental sounds.
- Consistently exaggerated or inappropriate responses to sounds that are neither threatening nor uncomfortably loud to the typical person.
- Abnormal lowered tolerance to sound.

The common thread to all these definitions is that people with hyperacusis find sounds in general intolerable, rather than specific sounds.

▌ Misophonia

This word was developed in 2001[1] and literally means a strong dislike or hatred of sound. The original intent was that this would represent a broad range of negative emotional responses to specific sounds irrespective of the sound level.

▌ Phonophobia

Phonophobia is a subsection of misophonia in which fear is the dominant emotion that is elicited by sound.

▌ Recruitment

Recruitment is a phenomenon seen in association with sensorineural hearing loss in which increasing sound intensity produces a greater than normal rise in perceived loudness.

▌ Acoustic shock

In the 1990s a cluster of symptoms was recognised in people working in call centres who had experienced sudden unexpected sounds through their headsets. The commonest symptoms were pain in or around the ear, hyperacusis, tinnitus and hypervigilance.[2] This symptom complex has subsequently been recognised in environments other than call centres.

▌ Altered definitions

The definition of misophonia has changed, partly as a result of input from patient groups, and is now often applied to a specific type of impaired sound tolerance, which is also known as selective (or soft) sound sensitivity syndrome, or simply 4S. This is characterised by emotions such as anger or disgust at sounds made by other people that often have an oral basis such as eating, throat clearing, yawning or breathing. Non-oral triggers are also reported including sounds such as toe tapping or joint cracking. Additionally, sufferers may be affected by visual stimuli such as someone fidgeting with their hair or swinging their legs while sitting. The negative emotions are often directed at specific people, often family members. A Dutch group has recently proposed that this condition should be recognised as a specific psychiatric condition.[3]

Alternative definitions

The classification described above is in common usage but an international working group has recently published a different set of definitions[4], consisting of loudness hyperacusis, annoyance hyperacusis, fear hyperacusis and pain hyperacusis. At the moment this is a proposal and it remains to be seen if it will usurp the existing classification.

EPIDEMIOLOGY

Prevalence

There is a paucity of evidence regarding the prevalence and incidence of hyperacusis. A study among adults in Sweden found a prevalence of 8.6%, whereas a Polish study found 15.2%. Hyperacusis is seen in all age groups and in a paediatric population a Brazilian study reported a prevalence of 3.2%. There is a strong association between hyperacusis and tinnitus; approximately 40% of people with significant tinnitus will report concomitant hyperacusis. In people who have hyperacusis as their primary complaint, up to 86% report that they also have tinnitus.

Comorbidities

Several medical conditions include hyperacusis as a symptom (**Table 30.1**). Some of these conditions, particularly those in the peripheral group, involve dysfunction of the facial nerve and hence potential loss of the protective stapedius reflex. Some patients with Lyme disease develop facial palsy but the majority do not. Hyperacusis can be seen in both groups, suggesting that Lyme disease may have both peripheral and central mechanisms for inducing hyperacusis.

Table 30.1. Medical conditions associated with hyperacusis, divided according to whether the underlying pathology is in the peripheral or central auditory system.

Peripheral	Central
● Facial nerve paresis including Bell's palsy and Ramsay Hunt syndrome ● Post stapedectomy ● Post grommet insertion ● Perilymph fistula ● Lyme disease	● Depression ● Migraine ● Head injury ● Post-traumatic stress disorder ● Lyme disease ● Fibromyalgia ● Williams syndrome ● Addison's disease

PATHOPHYSIOLOGY

As described above, some cases of hyperacusis seem to be caused by loss of the protective stapedius reflex. Such cases are rare. Various theories have been developed to explain the other cases:

● Increased central auditory gain as a plasticity response to reduced input from the ear.
● Increased central neural synchrony. Spontaneous neural activity in the auditory cortex is normally random. When the peripheral

auditory system is damaged, spontaneous cortical activity tends to become synchronised and there is speculation that this can give rise to tinnitus and can also alter the perception of sound intensity and hence give rise to hyperacusis.

- Reorganisation of the cortical auditory map. When the peripheral auditory system is damaged, one change seen in the auditory cortex is that neurons that received inputs from parts of the cochlea that have been damaged tune in to the nearest adjacent frequency input that is still active. This results in overrepresentation of frequencies adjacent to areas of damage and increased neural activity at those frequencies. It has been suggested that this produces hyperacusis.
- Failure of the medial olivocochlear efferent system, which is a descending neural pathway from the brain to the cochlea and exerts an inhibitory effect on the outer hair cells within

the cochlea. Impairment of this negative feedback process could generate hyperacusis.
- Dysfunction of serotonin pathways in the central auditory system. Many of the conditions seen as comorbidities of hyperacusis, including migraine, post-traumatic stress disorder and depression, have been postulated to be due to abnormalities within serotonin pathways. It has therefore been suggested that hyperacusis is a member of the same family of disorders.
- Dysfunction of gamma-aminobutyric acid inhibitory pathways in the central auditory system. This is another proposed mechanism by which normal negative feedback processes could become impaired.

All of these suggestions are at the hypothetical stage and there is no definite scientific proof for any of them. It is quite possible that there may be more than one mechanism for hyperacusis.

CLINICAL PRESENTATION/DIAGNOSIS

▐ History

When taking a clinical history from a hyperacusis patient, the clinician should try to ascertain what type of impaired sound tolerance is present. In addition to general questions regarding the auditory system, the clinician should also address the impact of the condition on daily life and the degree to which the person is avoiding sound. Other areas to cover include symptoms of potential comorbid conditions such as Lyme disease, migraine or depression.

▐ Examination

Clinical examination of hyperacusis patients is usually normal but it is important to check both the ears and cranial nerve function.

▐ Audiometry

Everyone presenting with hyperacusis should have an appropriate hearing test, usually a pure tone audiogram. This needs to be done carefully as by the nature of their condition, people with

hyperacusis are very wary of any form of test that involves exposure to sound.

Assessing tolerance to sound by measuring loudness discomfort levels (LDLs) can be useful in defining the extent of the problem and monitoring treatment but risks causing distress to the patient due to the levels of sound involved. If this test is proposed, it should be thoroughly explained and the patient should be offered the opportunity to decline the investigation. Testing the stapedius reflex involves significant sound levels and should be avoided unless there is a compelling clinical reason to proceed.

▐ Imaging

It may be desirable to undertake medical imaging of hyperacusis patients, particularly if there is associated asymmetric hearing or asymmetric tinnitus. The usual modality in this situation is MRI but it should be remembered that this is a very noisy investigation. As with LDL testing, the patient should be carefully counselled prior to testing.

Haematological

It is unusual for blood tests to be required in the investigation of hyperacusis unless the clinical history suggests a condition such as Lyme disease, in which case the appropriate serological test should be requested.

Questionnaires

Two questionnaire tools have been developed for use with hyperacusis patients but neither of these has yet been validated in an English speaking population. There is also a rating scale based on the impact of hyperacusis on activities of daily living – the multiple activity scale for hyperacusis (MASH).

MANAGEMENT

If the clinical history, examination and testing have identified a specific cause for the hyperacusis, this should be addressed.

Self-help

An online patient support forum is available at http://www.hyperacusis.net.

Counselling and general support

Many people with hyperacusis feel that they are disbelieved and that no one else has similar problems. Sufferers often describe hyperacusis as a hidden disability. Simple explanation and reassurance is often helpful. This can be undertaken as a standalone process or as part of a structured management paradigm (see Structured treatment programmes, below). Counselling should include advice about appropriate hearing protection measures. Many people with hyperacusis adopt fear-avoidance behaviour and keep away from sound, making their lives ever quieter. Although this seems like common sense, it is counter-productive as the absence of sound in the environment causes increased central auditory gain. Wearing hearing protection devices is sensible when in hazardous noise but use at other times should be avoided.

Sound therapy

Reintroducing sound to people with hyperacusis is generally beneficial and several techniques are employed. At home, and particularly at night time in the bedroom, environmental sound generators can be used. During the daytime when the person wishes to move outside the house, wide-band sound generators, which are worn in the ear, produce low levels of sound in an attempt to improve tolerance. Such devices also reduce contrast between background sound and the sounds that are not well-tolerated. Such devices can be used either with a continuous very low level of sound in a process known as recalibration or with slowly increasing sound level in a process known as desensitisation. There has also been some research looking at the use of hearing aids, which are set up so that their output cannot exceed certain limits. The upper limit can then be slowly increased as the hyperacusis improves. Some patients with hyperacusis feel unable to wear devices in their ears, in which case other techniques can be utilised such as wearing headphones loosely around the neck connected to an MP3 player.

Structured treatment programmes

Various attempts have been made to combine counselling and sound therapy in a structured process. Such modalities include tinnitus retraining therapy (TRT) and hyperacusis activities therapy (HAT).

Psychological treatments

Standard psychological management techniques, particularly cognitive behavioural therapy (CBT)[5], have been utilised with some success in hyperacusis.

CONCLUSION

Our understanding of hyperacusis and other disorders of sound tolerance is very much in its infancy. Little is known about the pathophysiology of such conditions and even the basic terminology remains contentious. Scientific interest has increased recently, partly as a result of pressure from patient groups, and an animal model of hyperacusis is being developed. Current treatment modalities are based on tinnitus treatments and their efficacy with regard to hyperacusis is largely unknown.

REFERENCES

1 Jastreboff MM, Jastreboff PJ (2001) Components of decreased sound tolerance: hyperacusis, misophonia, phonophobia. *ITHS News Lett* **2**:5–7.

2 McFerran DJ, Baguley DM (2007) Acoustic shock. *J Laryngol Otol* 13:133–134.

3 Ferreira GM, Harrison BJ, Fontenelle LF (2013) Hatred of sounds: misophonic disorder or just an underreported psychiatric symptom? *Ann Clin Psychiatry* **25(4)**:271–274.

4 Tyler RS, Pienkowski M, Rojas Roncancio E *et al.* (2014) A review of hyperacusis and future directions: Part I. Definitions and manifestations. *Am J Audiol* **23**:402–419.

5 Jüris L, Andersson G, Larsen HC *et al.* (2014) Cognitive behaviour therapy for hyperacusis: a randomized controlled trial. *Behav Res Ther* **54**:30–37.

31

AUDITORY PROCESSING DISORDER

Nicholas A. Quinn & Richard K. Gurgel

Contents

INTRODUCTION

Hearing is a complex process that requires the ability to detect sound waves via the peripheral auditory system (outer, middle and inner ear structures) and the ability of the central nervous system (CNS) to process the subsequent electrical impulses sent from the inner ear. The portion of hearing governed by the CNS is termed 'auditory processing', which is defined by the American Speech-Language-Hearing Association as the 'perceptual processing of auditory information in the CNS and the neurobiological activity that underlies that processing and gives rise to electrophysiological auditory potentials'.[1]

The diagnosis of (central) auditory processing disorder [(C)APD] is made when a patient has difficulty hearing that cannot be accounted for by peripheral hearing loss or other cognitive deficits. Patients with APD typically have difficulty in sound localisation, auditory discrimination (i.e. hearing in background noise), pattern recognition, temporal aspects of audition and auditory performance in competing acoustic signals. This causes functional impairments in listening, learning and spoken language comprehension and development.[1]

AETIOLOGY

The underlying aetiology of APD is diverse and not completely understood. It may result from degenerative disease, neurotoxic drugs, a seizure disorder or primary central auditory nervous system (CANS) lesions to name a few examples, although most

patients have no identifiable structural pathology. The heterogeneous nature of the underlying pathology underscores the fact that an APD may arise from dysfunction at any level of the auditory processing pathway. APD may be congenital or acquired and thus diagnosed at any age. There is, however, a tendency to focus efforts of research and diagnosis towards children given the potential for delays in learning and language development during formative years. Currently, the prevalence of APD in the paediatric population has been estimated at 3–10%.[2] There is evidence to support an association between APD and other developmental disorders, especially specific language impairment, dyslexia and attention-deficit hyperactivity disorder, which are also primarily diagnosed in the paediatric population. If one of these diagnoses is made, the clinician should strongly consider investigation for APD and vice versa. While APD may co-exist with other disorders, it is not necessarily the result of those disorders; to accurately diagnose APD there must be a demonstrable deficit at the level of the CANS that is not attributable to higher order cognitive deficits.

ASSESSMENT

Suspicion for APD should be raised when a patient has a history of functional impairment in learning, reading and language development or difficulty in noisy listening environments. History is a critical portion of the assessment provided by the patient, family members, teachers or employers. Symptoms can be quite subtle and are often combined with other comorbid sensory, behavioural or developmental disorders; consequently, early evaluation by a multidisciplinary team is crucial. Investigations to screen for related disorders should be performed if a diagnosis is not already known or ruled out. This includes testing for cognitive defects, language proficiency, speech intelligibility, peripheral hearing loss and other medical issues. This ensures that any comorbid conditions are also discovered and adequately treated to optimise patient outcomes.

A flow diagram for an initial patient evaluation is shown in **Figure 31.1**. While the flowchart is meant to convey the key elements of an approach to patients with APD, it is important to note that there is no gold standard or single diagnostic test to detect APD, so variations from this simplified algorithm may exist in clinical practice. The most recent recommendation from the American Academy of Audiology emphasises individualisation of testing based on individual patient history.[3] In almost all cases, initial investigations include pure tone audiometry, tympanometry, speech recognition thresholds and word recognition scores.[4] Further information is obtained through a combination of behavioural and physiological testing measures. To this end, there are a large number of tests available to the audiologist; broadly, they include the following: dichotic tests, monaural low-redundancy speech tests, temporal processing tests, binaural interaction tests and electrophysiological tests. (Refer to **Table 31.1** for further details of available tests.) The clinician will choose from these tests depending on the deficient areas each individual patient expresses.

MANAGEMENT

Once the diagnosis of APD has been made, treatment should be started immediately, especially for paediatric patients to take advantage of the inherent neuroplasticity of the developing child's brain. Depending on the specific deficits identified, therapy is individualised for each patient, but in all cases should be multimodal in nature and delivered by a multidisciplinary team in the same way the diagnosis was made. Typically, this team includes audiologists, speech and language therapists, teachers, psychologists and parents. Therapy is generally comprised of three broad approaches: environmental modification, skills remediation and compensatory strategies.

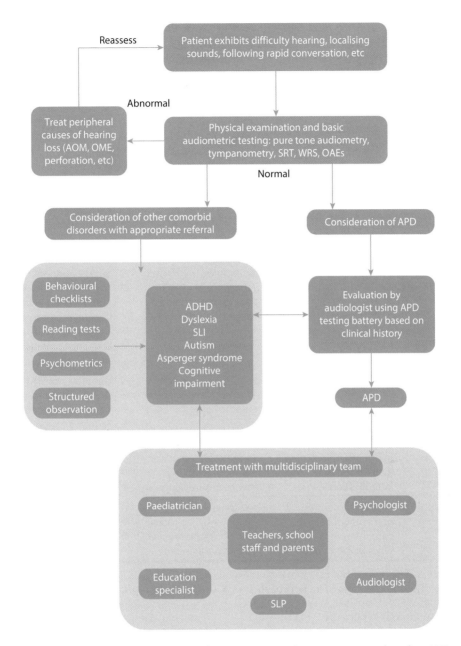

Figure 31.1. Flow diagram for initial patient evaluation. APD, auditory processing disorder; SRT, speech recognition threshold; WRS, word recognition score; OAEs, otoacoustic emissions; AOM, acute otitis media; OME, otitis media with effusion; ADHD, attention-deficit hyperactivity disorder; SLI, specific language impairment; SLP, speech language pathologist.

● Environmental modification typically aims to improve signal-to-noise ratio for the listener with APD. Environmental modifications may include moving students near the front of the classroom, reducing background noise, utilising assistive listening devices, gaining the attention of the listener before speaking and speaking more slowly.

Table 31.1. Auditory processing disorder diagnostic testing options.

Test category	Assesses	Method	Examples
Dichotic tests	CNS integration of information presented in both ears	Distinct stimuli presented to both ears simultaneously; listener's goal is to process both stimuli or to ignore one ear only	• Dichotic digits • Staggered spondaic word • SCAN competing words • SCAN competing sentences • Synthetic sentence identification with contralateral competing message • Competing sentences test • Dichotic consonant vowel task • Dichotic rhyme test
Monaural low-redundancy speech tests	Ability to fill in missed sounds including words, syllables or phonemes	Sounds are presented to only one ear, modified to reduce signal redundancy by filtering out a frequency or adding background noise	• High-pass filtered speech • Low-pass filtered speech • SCAN filtered words • SCAN auditory figure ground • Synthetic sentence identification with ipsilateral competing message • Speech-in-noise • U-6 time-compressed speech
Temporal processing tests	Pattern perception and ability to distinguish sounds relative to temporal presentation	Listener must discriminate sounds based on sequence or temporal order	• Pitch pattern • Duration pattern • Gaps-in-noise • Random gap detection test • Auditory fusion test – revised
Binaural interaction tests	Integration of binaural information, including localisation and lateralisation	Similar stimuli are presented to each ear non-simultaneously; listener must distinguish	• Rapidly alternating speech perception • Binaural fusion test • Masking level difference
Electrophysiological tests	Integrity of inner ear and cortical central nervous system physiological function	Uses specialised equipment/electrodes; does not require active listener participation	• Auditory brainstem response • Middle latency response • Cortical evoked potentials

● Remediation is also known as auditory training and seeks to directly reduce the APD through methods such as phoneme discrimination, auditory closure training and temporal training. To describe each of these briefly, phoneme discrimination involves detecting the differences between similar words that differ by one phoneme, the smallest significant units of spoken language that give a word its specific meaning (e.g. pat vs. pet or lease vs. leash). Auditory closure training is a technique that utilises the patients knowledge, vocabulary and experiences to fill in missing or distorted auditory information in order to complete a spoken word (e.g. "bana_a"). Temporal training focuses on the sequencing of words/sounds, which can be problematic with more rapid speech. Earobics™ is a popularly used software program among providers that combines many of the above mentioned activities into interactive games focused on children in their early years.[3]

- Compensatory strategies focus on strengthening higher order cognitive areas to provide better functional outcomes, even if the APD if not fully resolved with remediation strategies. This includes training in active listening, context-based vocabulary building and assertiveness training (speaking up when the message was not heard), and metamemory such as the use of mnemonics or repeating back to the speaker what was heard to improve memory.

Through a combination of these strategies, patients should develop the ability to communicate and listen more effectively at school, home and work. Ultimately, the goal is to improve functional outcomes, but in order to track progress most audiologists will use objective scores, which may be derived by repeating the same tests as those used in the diagnosis of APD. Treatment yields a favourable prognosis with anecdotal evidence of improvement per parents/family as well as statistically significant improvements on objective auditory and language testing as evidenced by small studies.[5] However, such large variations exist between interventions that there remains a lack of robust data that can be generalised to the APD population as a whole until further research is performed.

REFERENCES

1 American Speech-Language-Hearing Association (2005) (Central) auditory processing disorders [Technical Report]. Available from www.asha.org/policy.

2 Witton C (2010) Childhood auditory processing disorder as a developmental disorder: the case for a multi-professional approach to diagnosis and management. *Int J Audiol* **49(2)**:83–87.

3 American Academy of Audiology (2010) *Clinical Practice Guidelines: Diagnosis, Treatment and Management of Children and Adults with Central Auditory Processing Disorder*. American Academy of Audiology, August 2010.

4 Emanuel DC, Ficca KN, Korczak P (2011) Survey of the diagnosis and management of auditory processing disorder. *Am J Audiol* **20**:48–60.

5 Sharma M, Purdy SC, Kelly AS (2012) A randomized controlled trial of interventions in school-aged children with auditory processing disorders. *Int J Audiol* **51**:506–518.

32 FUTURE THERAPIES

Mahmood F. Bhutta

Contents

INTRODUCTION

Recent years have witnessed tremendous advances in biological techniques, pharmaceutical methods and materials science. These advances have enabled a number of potential new therapies for hearing loss, some of which are outlined below.

BALLOON EUSTACHIAN TUBOPLASTY

Narrowing of the Eustachian tube may be one factor in the perpetuation of chronic otitis media. Balloons have been developed to dilate the cartilaginous portion of the Eustachian tube. Initial results of this treatment are encouraging, demonstrating reversal of long-standing tympanic membrane retraction. At present this treatment has been used on cohorts with a variety of middle ear diseases. To clarify the role of this new treatment, future studies will need to employ better definitions of disease and use patient reported outcome measures.

HYPOXIA SIGNALLING IN CHRONIC OTITIS MEDIA

Work from my own laboratory has shown that the chronically inflamed middle ear is hypoxic. Hypoxia is a common finding in chronically inflamed microenvironments and molecular signalling resulting from hypoxia can contribute to inflammation. Studies in mouse models of chronic otitis media show that antagonising hypoxia signalling with systemically administered vascular endothelial growth factor receptor (VEGFR) inhibitors leads to downregulation of inflammation and moderation of hearing loss. A technique for local delivery of molecular therapies to the middle ear will be needed before they can enter clinical trials.

TISSUE ENGINEERED MIDDLE EAR MUCOSA

In persistent chronic otitis media the middle ear gas pocket can collapse, leading to poor hearing. Current evidence suggests that ventilation of the middle ear is reliant on transmucosal gas exchange in the posterosuperior mesotympanum and mastoid, assisted by periodic opening of the Eustachian tube. This mucosa can be damaged by chronic inflammation or by surgery. Studies in rabbits have shown that healthy middle ear mucosa can be explanted, grown on tissue scaffolds and then reimplanted, and that this mucosa is functional and can contribute to ventilation of the middle ear (at least in the short term). The challenge in patients with chronic otitis media is that the mucosa is unhealthy, and tissue engineering of diseased mucosa may prove not to be as successful.

IMPROVED RESOLUTION OF COCHLEAR IMPLANTS

Contemporary cochlear implants are limited in their auditory resolution because they use electrodes positioned some distance from the auditory nerve. This leads to rather indiscrete stimulation, and a limitation on the number of electrode arrays that can be employed. More discrete methods for stimulation are being explored, including intra-nerve electrodes and optical stimulation with lasers.

MOLECULAR THERAPY FOR SYNDROMIC HEARING LOSS

A large number of syndromes are associated with sensorineural hearing loss (SNHL), and advances in genetic sequencing have enabled the identification of the causal genetic mutation in such syndromes, even on an individual patient basis. This opens an opportunity to target the genetic defect to prevent, or even reverse, hearing loss.

Usher syndrome is characterised by both blindness and progressive hearing loss. In a mouse model of Usher syndrome, a single dose of RNA designed to inhibit the defective *Ush1c* gene has been delivered to the cochlea. When given to neonatal mice, this therapy prevented degeneration of hair cells and protected low frequency hearing. It is likely this therapy will soon progress to clinical trials, and if successful, this approach could be emulated to explore treatment of a number of other syndromes associated with progressive SNHL.

MOLECULAR THERAPY FOR PRESBYACUSIS AND NOISE-INDUCED HEARING LOSS

Excitotoxicity is thought to be a key mechanism in both noise-induced hearing loss and in presbyacusis. Overstimulation of hair cells leads to release of adenosine triphosphate, calcium and free radicals. Treatment with antagonists of some of these pathways, in particular anti-oxidants, have shown promise in animal studies, and some are now being trialled in man. Liposomes, viral vectors or nanoparticles may enable local delivery of these drugs to the cochlea, which will significantly enhance their therapeutic potential.

HAIR CELL REGENERATION

An alternative strategy for auditory hair cell degeneration is to use regeneration. Several strategies have been reported. The first is to induce proliferation of mature hair cells by deleting genes that normally regulate the cell cycle. However, this approach has shown limited success in animals models, and there are concerns that such proliferation could proceed uncontrolled. Another approach is the conversion of cochlear supporting cells into hair cells, in particular exploiting overexpression of the gene *Atoh1*, a known regulator of hair cell differentiation that has shown promise in animal trials and is now entering human trials. The final approach is to use stem cells, either undifferentiated embryonic stem cells or stem cells from within the cochlea. Stem cells have been successfully induced to differentiate into primitive cochlear hair cells, but these cells show little evidence of integration with auditory neurons, meaning they are likely to be non-functional. There is much potential for hair cell regeneration as a new treatment, particularly for presbyacusis, but achieving clinically important results may still be a distant goal.

FURTHER READING

Sudhoff H, Bhutta M (2014) (eds.) *Recent Advances in Otolaryngology, Volume 9*. JP Medical Ltd., London.

INDEX